Single Surgical Procedures 12

A Colour Atlas of

Operations on the Internal Carotid Artery

H.H.G. Eastcott
MS, FRCS, FRCOG, Hon. FACS, Hon. FRACS
Consulting Surgeon,
St Mary's Hospital,
London

Wolfe Medical Publications Ltd

Published by Wolfe Medical Publications Ltd, 1984
Printed by Royal Smeets Offset b.v.,
Weert, Netherlands
ISBN 0 7234 1023 2
ISSN 0264–8695

This book is one of the titles in the series of Wolfe Single Surgical Procedures, a series which will eventually cover some 200 titles.

If you wish to be kept informed of new additions to the series and receive details of our other titles, please write to Wolfe Medical Publications Ltd, Wolfe House, 3 Conway Street, London W1P 6HE.

A few of the other titles in print and in preparation in the Single Surgical Procedures series

Parotidectomy
Traditional Meniscectomy
Inguinal Hernias & Hydroceles in Infants and Children
Surgery for Pancreatic & Associated Carcinomata
Subtotal Thyroidectomy
Boari Bladder-Flap Procedure
Treatment of Carpal Tunnel Syndrome
Anterior Resection of Rectum
Seromyotomy for Chronic Duodenal Ulcer
Resection of Aortic Aneurysm
Modified Radical Mastectomy
Total Gastrectomy
Ileo-Rectal Anastomosis
Pre-Prosthetic Oral Surgery
Surgery for Undescended Testes
Techniques of Nerve Grafting and Repair
Surgery for Dupuytren's Contracture
Athrodesis of the Ankle
Surgery for Congenital Dislocation of the Hip
Common Operations of the Foot
Femoral and Tibial Osteotomy
Maxillo-Facial Traumatology
Surgery for Chondromalacia Patellae
Stabilisation for Extensive Spinal Injury
Spondylolisthesis
Laminectomy
Gall Bladder Cholecystectomy
Repair of Prolapsed Rectum
Proctocolectomy
Resection of Oesophagus
Splenectomy
Thyroid Lobectomy
Hirschprung's Disease
Extra-cranial and Intra-cranial Anastomosis
Anterior Nephrectomy
Bladder Augmentation
Caecocystoplasty
Hiatus Hernia
Total Gastrectomy
Billroth 1 Gastrectomy
Billroth 2 Gastrectomy
Abdominal Incisions
Thoracotomy
Chronic Pancreatitis Operation
Surgery for Strictures in Common Bile Duct
Biliary Enteric Anastomosis
Partial Hepatectomy
Splenectomy
Right Hemicolectomy
Appendicectomy
Incisional Hernia
Lung Lobectomy
Lung Removal
Gastric Reconstruction
Surgery for Lymphoedema
Kidney Transplants
Liver Transplant
Pancreas Transplant
Dialysis Techniques
Surgery for Thoracic Outlet
Haemorrhoids
Abdominoperineal Resection of Rectum
Rectosigmoid Resection
Non-resectional Surgery for Multiple Bowel Stenosis
Surgery for Anorectal Incontinence
Craniotomy
Parathyroidectomy
Arterial Injuries
Arterial Bypass Grafts in Leg
Visceral Vascular Occlusion
Varicose Veins under Local Anaesthesia
Aortofemoral Bypass
Aortoiliac Disobliteration
Technique of Small Vessel Repair
Technique of Nerve Grafting and Repair
Microsurgery Techniques
Reimplantation of Ureters
Pyloric Stenosis in Children
Cleft Palate Surgery
Anorectal Malformation
Amputations of the Lower Limb
Anterolateral Decompression
Spinal Fusion
Scoliosis
Spinal Fusion for Low Back Pain
Anterior Fusion of Cervical Spine
Recurrent Dislocation of Shoulder
Joint Replacement of Elbow
Joint Replacement of Wrist and Hand
Operative Fixation of Fractures of the Forearm
Joint Replacement at the Hip
Joint Replacement at the Knee
Arthrodesis of the Knee
Triple Arthrodesis
Discogram Surgery – Lumbar Disc
Amputations of the Upper Limb and Hand
Plastering Techniques
Operations for Peripheral Nerve
Compression Syndromes
Techniques of Tendon Transfer in the Upper Limb
Arthrodesis of the Wrist
Reconstructive Procedures of the Thumb
Flexor Tendon Repair and Grafting
Minor Operative Procedures
Technique of Arthroscopy of the Knee
Management of Fresh Ligamentous Injuries of the Knee

Contents

Dedication

To Bobbie

Acknowledgements

I am grateful to Dr Peter Cardew and the other members of the Audiovisual Department, St Mary's Hospital Medical School for the clinical and operative photographs used in this book, and to Dr David Sutton for the arteriograms. Dr James Bull provided those shown in Figures **79** and **80** and Dr Michael Ashby the retinal photograph (Figure **3**). The main sequence of carotid body excision views was kindly provided by Miss Averil Mansfield, to whom I am most indebted for this skilful demonstration of the technique that we both use. I have been much helped by Dr David Thomas, upon whose skill and good judgement in the neurological assessment and decision-taking so much has depended. My special thanks are due to Dr Peter Knight for his dedicated anaesthetic and early postoperative care. Some of the views in the endarterectomy series were taken at an operation performed by my then Senior Registrar Mr Andrew Lamerton, who also made the operative sketch from which I have drawn Figure **96**. The non-invasive investigation of most of the endarterectomy cases was carried out in the Irvine Vascular Laboratory, St Mary's Hospital, under the direction of Professor Andrew Nicolaides, to whom I am so much in debt for all his help with these and other cases during the past 12 years. The duplex seen in Figure **6**, by Mr Michael Williams is a good example of the continuing progress in this pioneer unit. Other pictures have been difficult to trace to source, so if any acknowledgement of these is lacking I am sorry, and would wish to thank these other colleagues for their part in making this book. Lastly, my sincere thanks to Wolfe Medical Publications for their advice and patient help during its preparation.

Introduction

The objective of most carotid operations is the removal of partially occlusive disease of the internal carotid sinus before either complete obstruction, or more often embolic detachment of unstable atheromatous material can cause a major hemiplegic stroke. Yet this tragedy may complicate the operation itself, and is the chief reason for the controversy that has long surrounded the subject, not only among neurologists, as to the clinical indications for surgery, or when to undertake the invasive investigations that must precede it; but also among vascular surgeons, over the various technical means by which they hope the catastrophe of perioperative stroke may be avoided. Since figures for combined stroke/mortality incidence vary between 2.5 and 25 per cent, and because complications do not appear to bear any general relationship to the use, or non-use of protective measures such as carotid shunting, the safety of carotid endarterectomy seems to depend more upon who is doing the operation than the protective measures adopted. This does not mean that shunting may now be abandoned, only that in some skilled hands it has proved to be unnecessary.

All experts agree that technical details, for example gentle handling of the thrombus-containing carotid bifurcation, close scrutiny for atheromatous remnants and first-class anaesthetic and recovery room care are essential for the safe conduct of these patients through this primarily preventive operation. It should not be embarked upon without special preparation and training in these principles. Its dangers partly arise from the deceptive simplicity and limited extent of the technique.

Other major hazards follow mistakes in case selection which mean that even though operative and anaesthetic skills should be equal to the well known problems and difficulties that arise in this work, success may be less than expected because of patient-related factors such as a recent stroke, labile hypertension, or active ischaemic heart disease.

These dangers may be hidden at the time of the preoperative clinical assessment, though nowadays they are often revealed by CT head scanning, which has become a routine investigation in most major centres, and by close attention to the state of the heart, which should be subjected to the same quality of medical review as in the patient under consideration for coronary surgery, including non-invasive studies and sometimes even coronary angiography as well, for modern experience has shown that acute myocardial infarction is one of the common causes of death after carotid endarterectomy as it is after most other peripheral vascular operations. If, at investigation, a serious coronary lesion is found, a decision must be taken on the relative priority of the two problems, to decide which operation should be performed first, or whether the two should be combined at a single session. Close cooperation with a consultant neurologist and a cardiologist is therefore essential.

The carotid lesion, its detection and its dangers

1

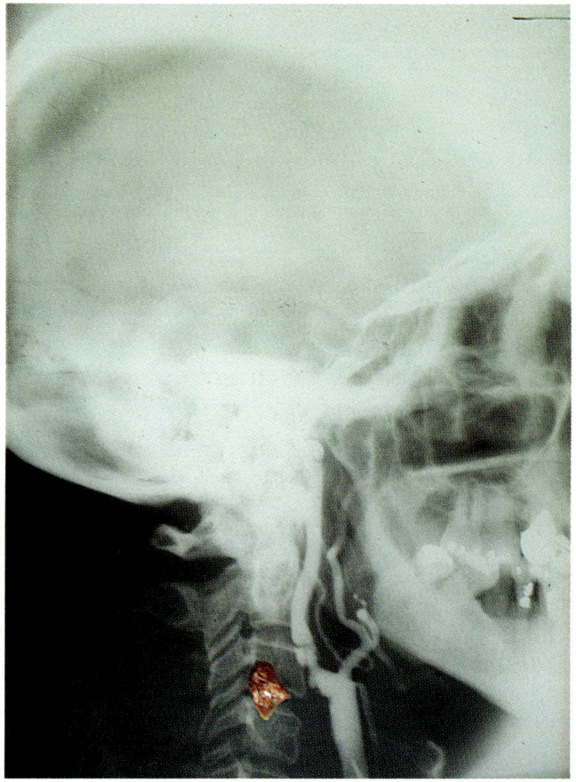

1 **Irregular stenosis of internal carotid.** An endarterectomy specimen and the arteriogram that detected the lesion. This is usually by selective transfemoral catheterisation, which also allows general views to be taken of the other major aortic arch branches.

2

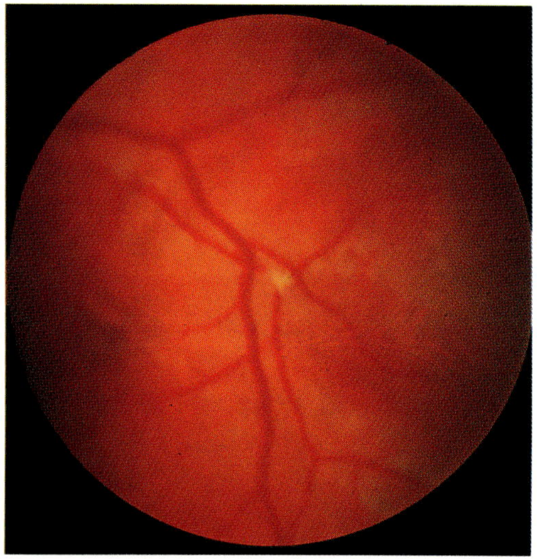

2 **Cholesterol retinal plaque.** A bright, shining body that has lodged at a bifurcation, supporting the diagnosis of ulcerating carotid atheroma.

3

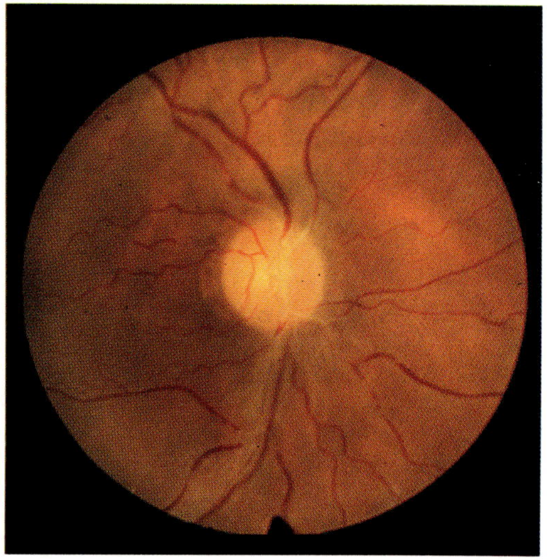

3 **Transient platelet embolism.** This is the probable mechanism of amaurosis fugax in carotid disease, and of most, if not all transient ischaemic hemisphere attacks.

4

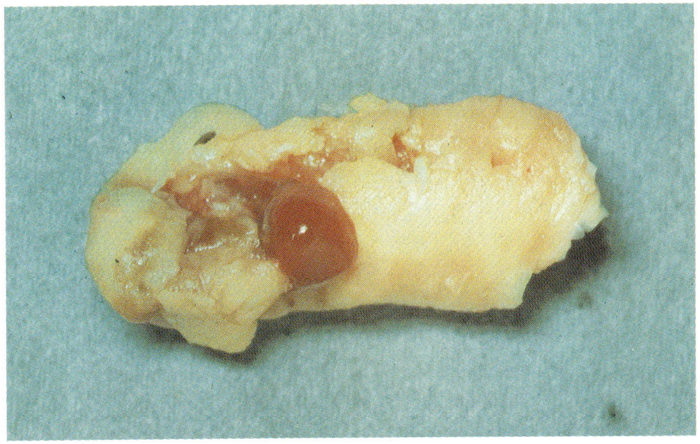

4 'The loaded gun'. Large, unstable rounded thrombus just beyond a carotid stenosis. Embolisation of such material would most probably occlude the blood supply to most of the motor area.

5

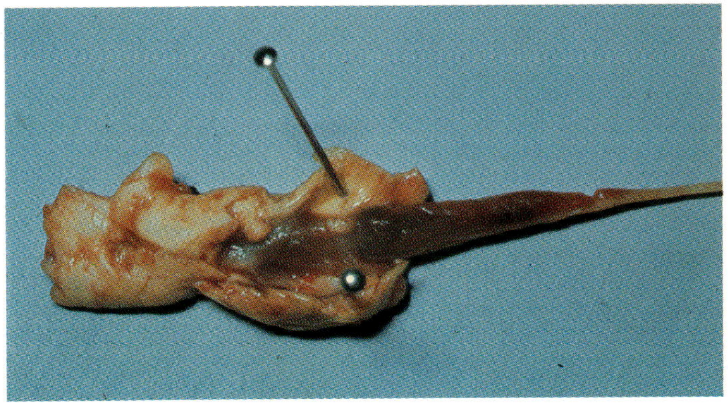

5 Progressive stable thrombus. From a doctor patient with a moderately severe, static left hemisphere defect, who after this operation made a prompt and almost complete recovery.

6

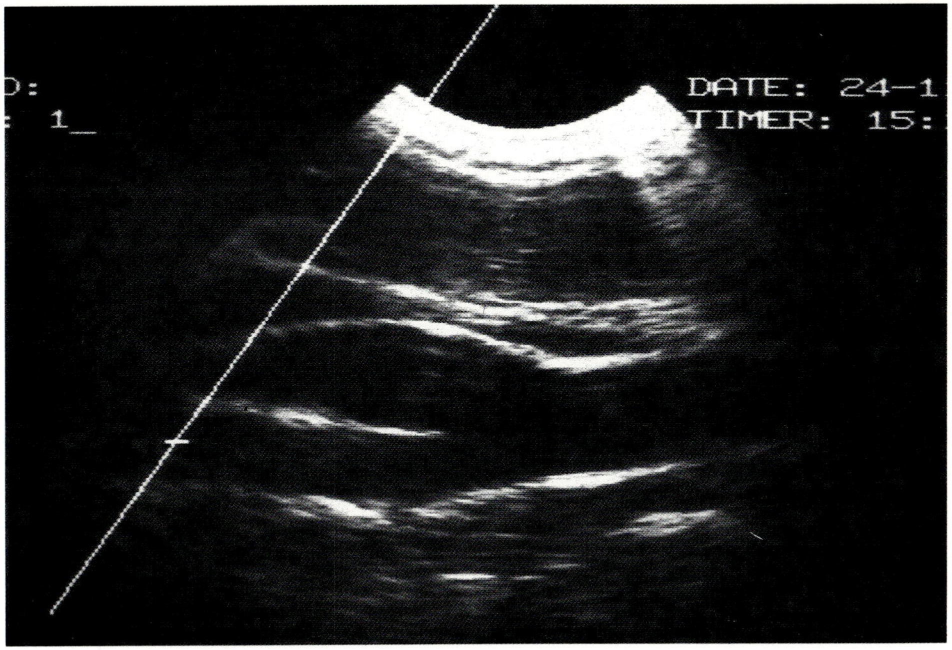

6 Duplex scanner. The present non-invasive diagnostic method of choice for use before arteriography in the investigation of transient hemisphere or retinal ischaemia. It provides both an image and a quantification of flow conditions at the point where the spot is directed. Its sensitivity (freedom from false negative results) and specificity (freedom from false positives) are high. The figure shows a normal carotid bifurcation with the sampling spot placed in the external carotid.

Indications for carotid endarterectomy

1 Recent, repeated transient ischaemic attacks affecting one cerebral hemisphere, or unilateral amaurosis fugax; with confirmed stenosis of the appropriate internal carotid sinus or of the common carotid bifurcation.

2 Mild, persistent neurological defect (not more recent than four weeks). Any large infarct of the affected hemisphere detected on computer tomographic (CT) scanning would bring this indication into question, also that described under 1 above.

3 Some patients with progressive or variable neurological defect, seen early and free from CT evidence of cerebral infarction.

4 Some patients with the indications described above in whom there is the need for a coronary bypass operation will need their carotid operation first.

5 Some patients with proven, severely stenotic or ulcerated carotid disease, yet free from neurological or ocular symptoms, for whom other major surgery is required. A carotid bruit on its own is not sufficient justification for a surgical programme. This would need non-invasive investigation, which, if it suggested that the stenosis was severe or ulcerated, could lead to angiography and consideration for surgery.

6 Asymptomatic disease of the type described under 5 above, in whom the other carotid has already been operated upon for symptomatic disease. This indication would not apply to the milder forms of carotid lesion, which are common and probably harmless in most instances.

Contraindications to carotid endarterectomy

1 Recent major stroke. There is a 40% operative mortality in such patients from haemorrhage into their cerebral infarct.

2 Most progressive neurological defects will similarly be worsened, especially those with CT evidence of infarction.

3 Second side operation, though often justified on the grounds mentioned above under 1 to 6 should not be undertaken sooner than 7 to 14 days after the first side.

4 'Tandem' stenosis of the distal portion of the internal carotid, unless smooth and regular, might form a source for middle cerebral embolism if the flow through it were to be suddenly increased by widening of the obstructed carotid sinus below.

5 Abdominal aortic aneurysm, if expanding, tender or otherwise actively symptomatic may need to take priority over an accompanying carotid lesion.

An illustrative case

A woman aged 60 underwent left carotid endarterectomy for a variable neurological defect three years before and sustained a mild right hand weakness. Two months before this arch aortogram and CT scan she developed further speech and right arm and leg impairment. The operated carotid has restenosed and the opposite one has silently occluded. An extensive left middle cerebral infarct was shown to be present. The patient was becoming progressively worse, so after careful neurological review the left carotid was reoperated, using an indwelling shunt and applying a vein patch graft. Immediately after operation she was found to be semistuporose with severely spastic right limbs, and died on the 16th postoperative day having become quadriplegic. Progressive recent stroke with occlusion of the opposite carotid should have contraindicated the operation.

7

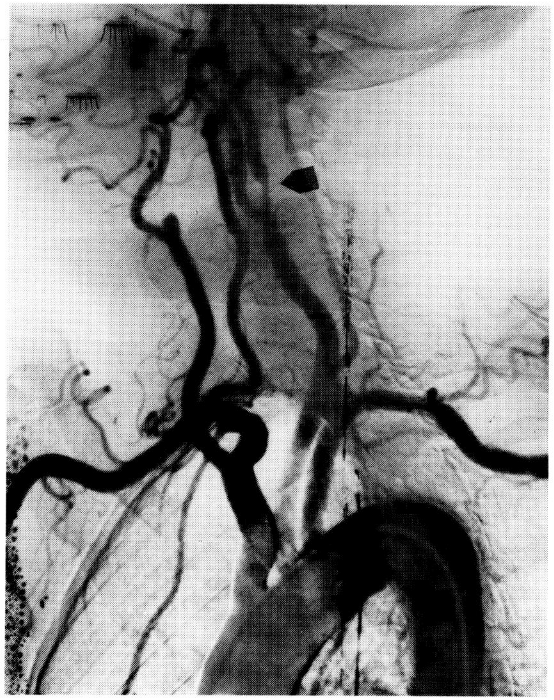

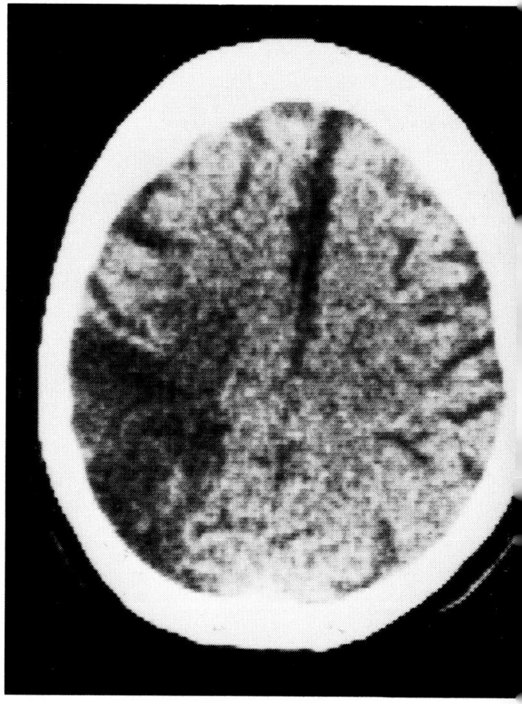

8
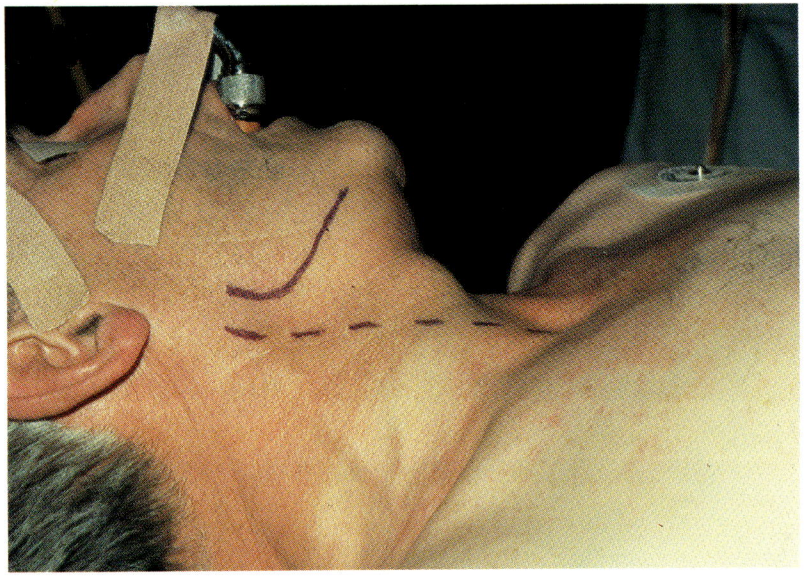

8 The patient is positioned with a small pad beneath the shoulders; general endotracheal anaesthesia is monitored using a radial artery line connected to a pressure transducer. Electrocardiographic surveillance is also essential. Electroencephalography if conveniently available in the theatre may give an early warning of impending stroke. Local analgesia by cervical plexus block with the patient conscious and cooperating can also give this information. Under such circumstances most surgeons would interrupt the procedure for the insertion of an indwelling carotid shunt.

9
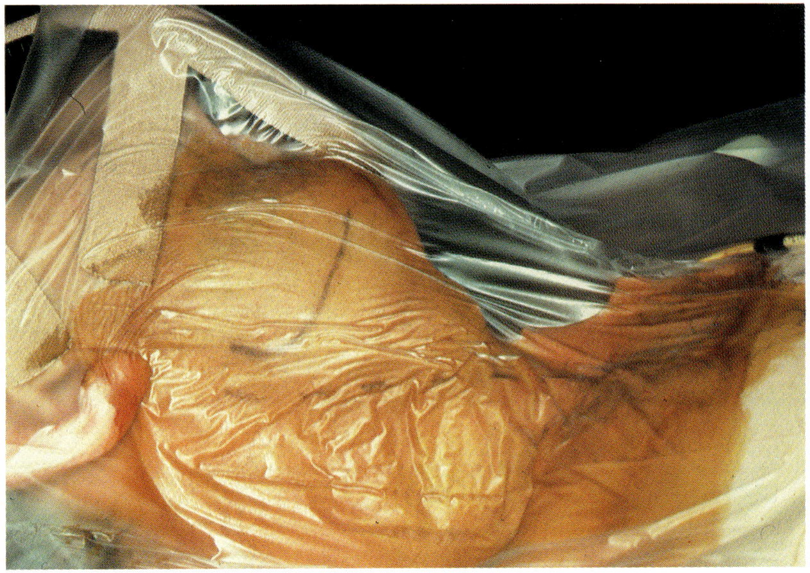

9 Adhesive sheeting over the marked operative area effectively screens it from nearby sources of potential contamination such as the ear, nose or the eye.

10

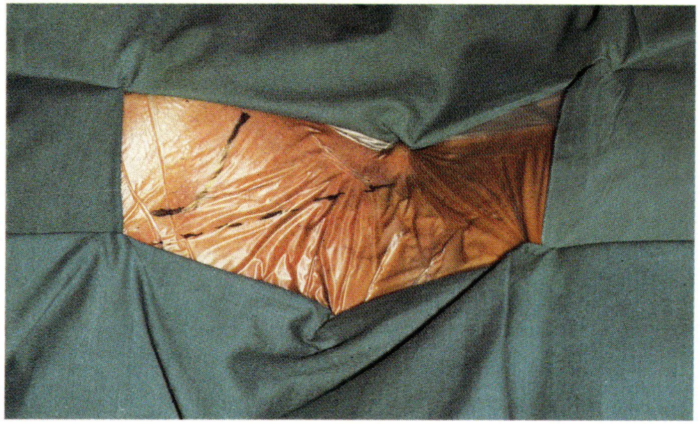

10 The wound is then draped so as to keep a clear view of the upper parotid area, where the distal internal carotid will later need to be fully exposed. The ear lobule is included in the field, for purposes of orientation and the correct placing of the incision.

11

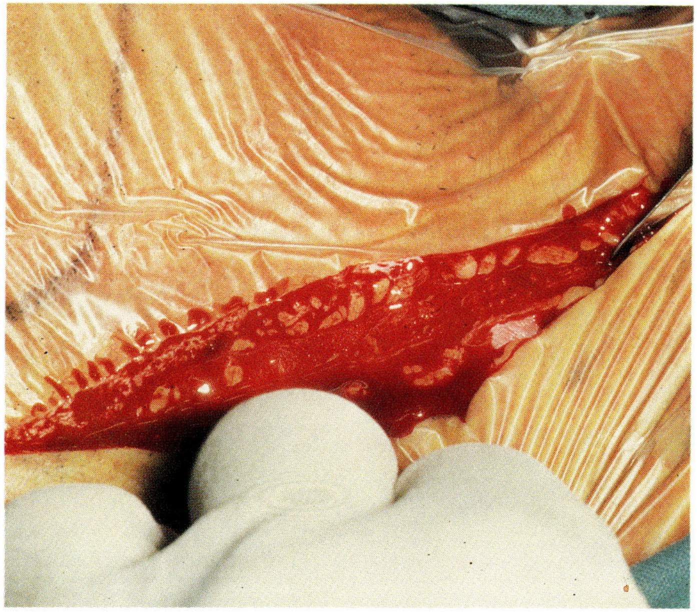

12

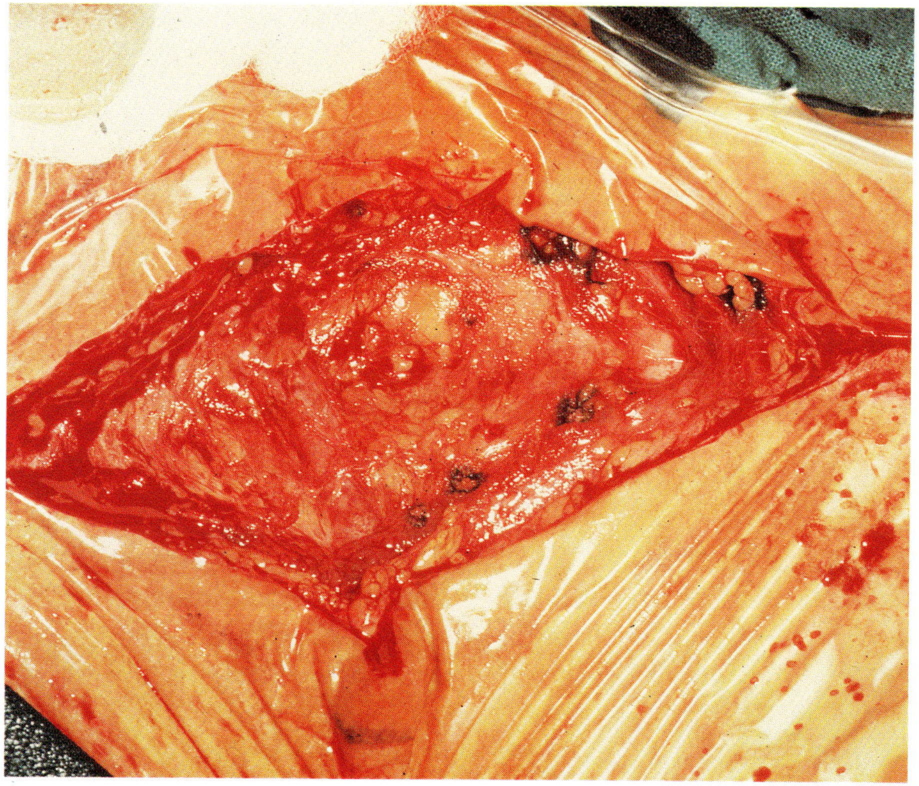

12 Division of the platysma muscle with the scalpel. Most carotid patients, having received aspirin before their operation, bleed rather freely from the superficial layers of the exposure.

11 The first skin incision is made along the anterior border of the sternomastoid muscle, centring on the carotid bifurcation, previously located on the arteriogram in its relation to the angle of the jaw. It is normally situated 2 or 3 cm below this level, seldom much higher, but often lower, sometimes well down in the neck. Keeping the upper end of the incision well back helps to avoid the cervical branch of the facial. The lower part of the incision should not approach the sternoclavicular joint, or a tight scar will result in this area.

13

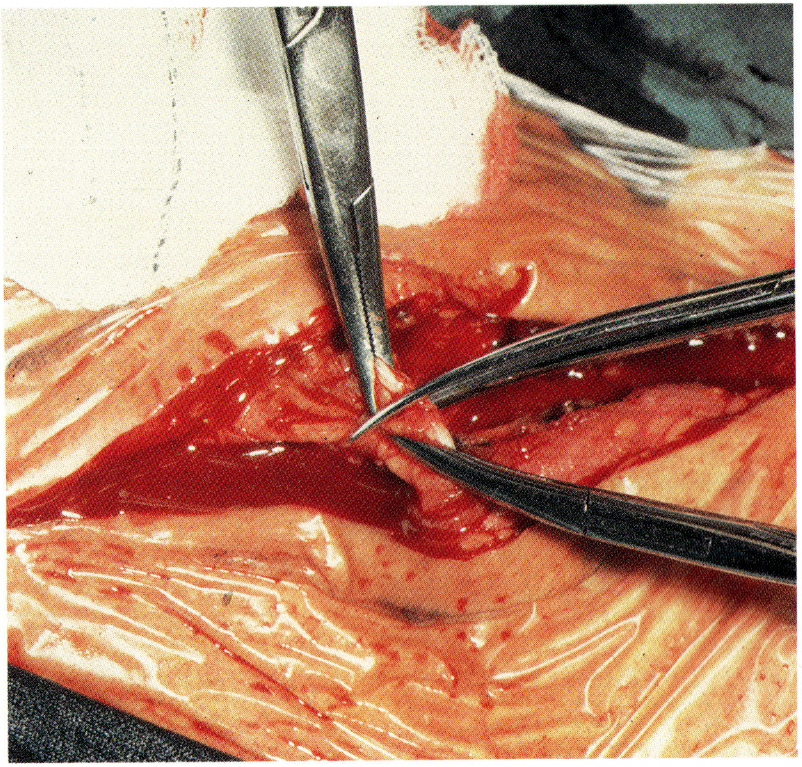

13 Ligation of a crossing cutaneous nerve and vessel. The greater auricular nerve lies in the upper part of the wound and should be avoided or preserved if at all possible. The anterior cutaneous, as here, must be divided to gain access. Diathermy should not be used for such situations; in fact it is best avoided altogether in this operation except for isolated minor bleeding points away from anatomical structures.

14

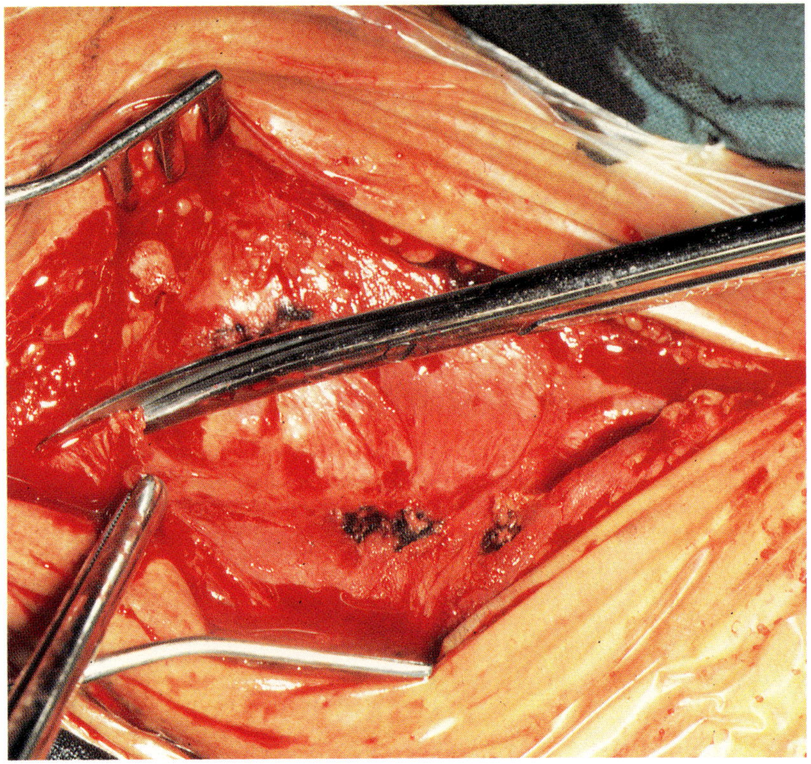

14 The deep fascia is divided using McIndoe's scissors, with Emmett's forceps in the left hand.

15

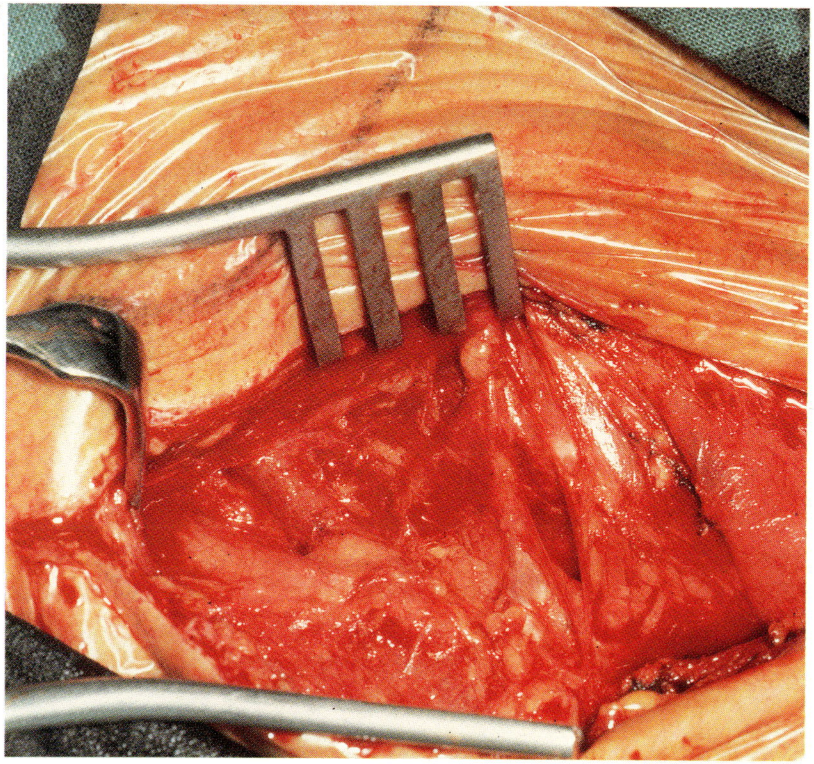

16

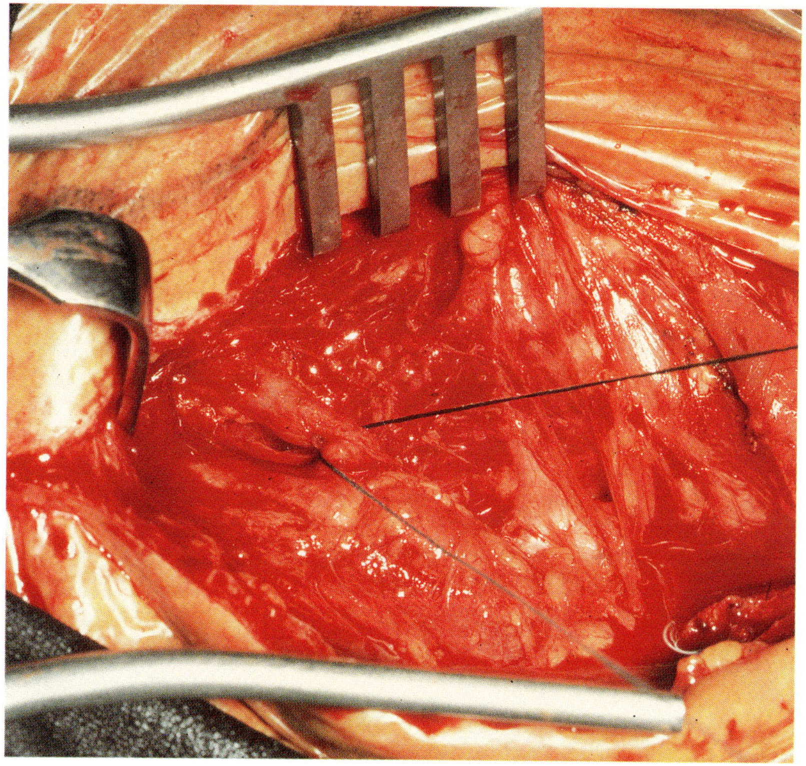

15 A West's self retaining retractor is inserted, the handles lying either below, or – if they are too high on the clavicle – they are placed above, as in this case. A Langenbeck's hand retractor at the upper end of the wound brings into view the prominence of the common facial vein, and helps also to control superficial oozing.

16 A 2/0 polyglycollic ligature is passed beneath the mobilised common facial vein.

17

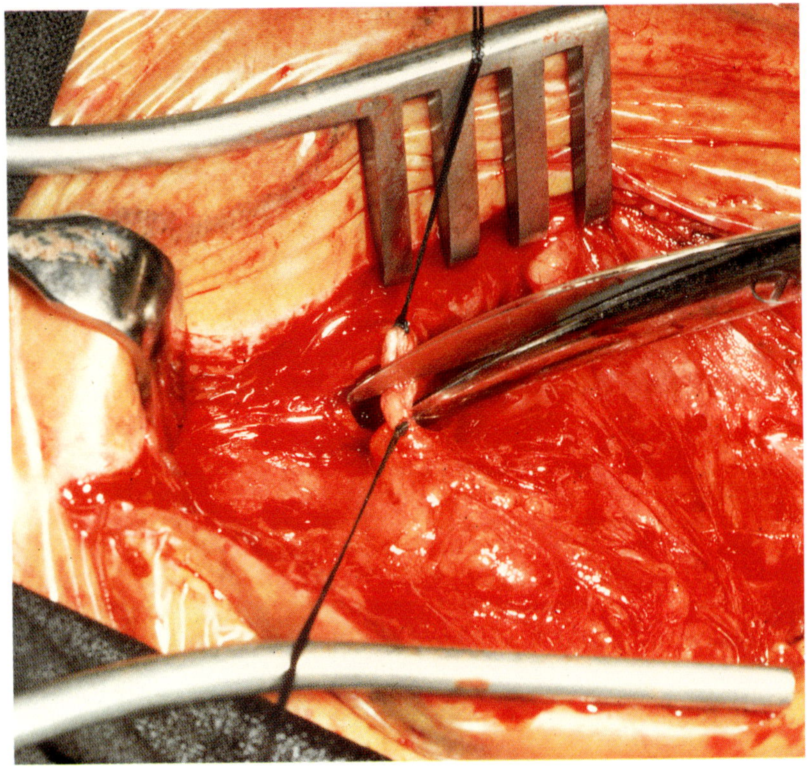

17 The common facial vein is divided between two ligatures.

18

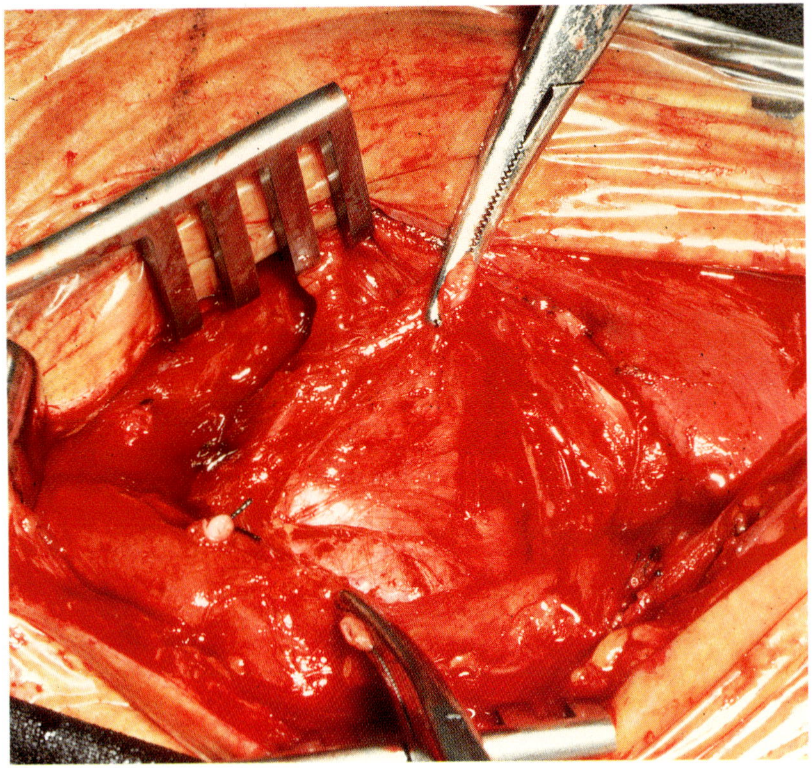

18 A second vein is clipped with Dunhill's artery forceps; gentle lateral traction on these gives us the first view of the carotid.

19

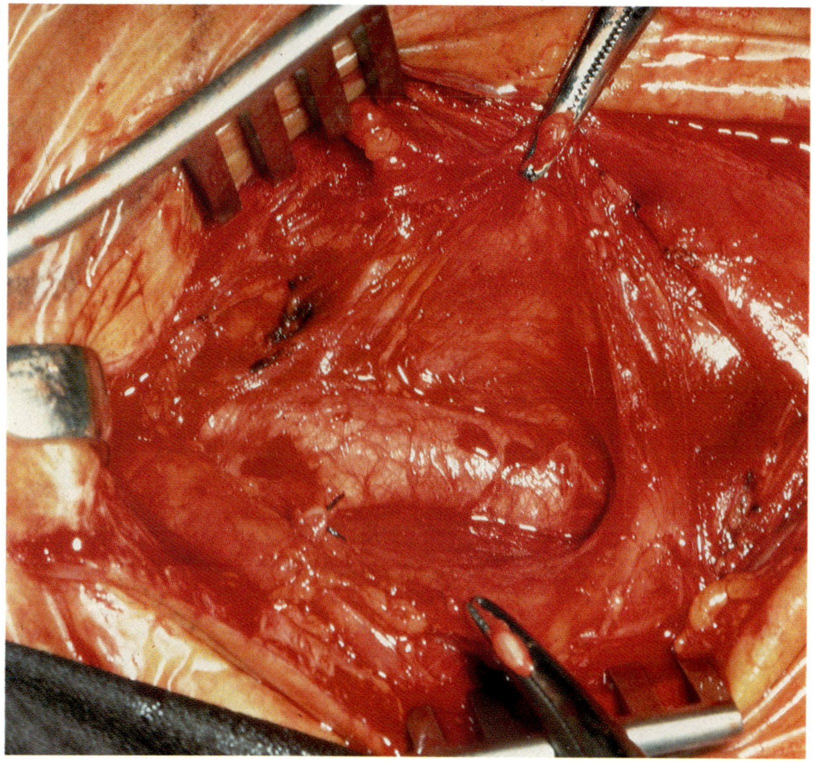

19 Further scissors dissection of this fascial plane has increased the carotid exposure. The origin of the superior thyroid artery can be seen anteriorly, identifying the external carotid not far away from the carotid bifurcation. In the words of my colleague, J. R. Kenyon, 'the tissues should be lifted off the carotid'.

20

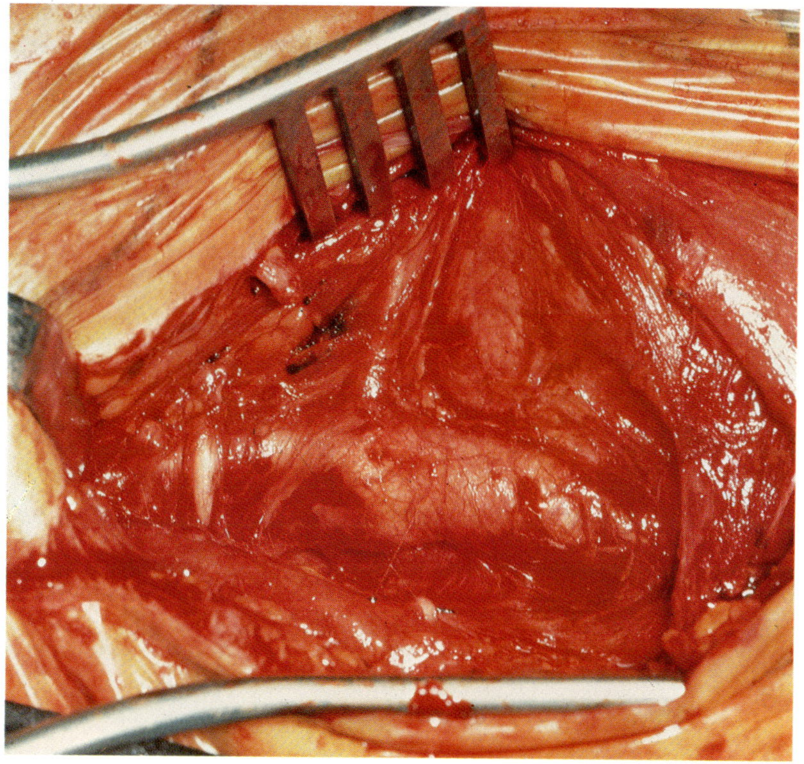

20 Cautious and gentle dissection in this plane exposes the hypoglossal nerve crossing the two carotids about a centimetre above the superior thyroid origin. No attempt is yet made to dissect further round the bifurcation. This is the most dangerous stage in the operation, when loose material within the stenosis may easily be embolised into the brain.

21

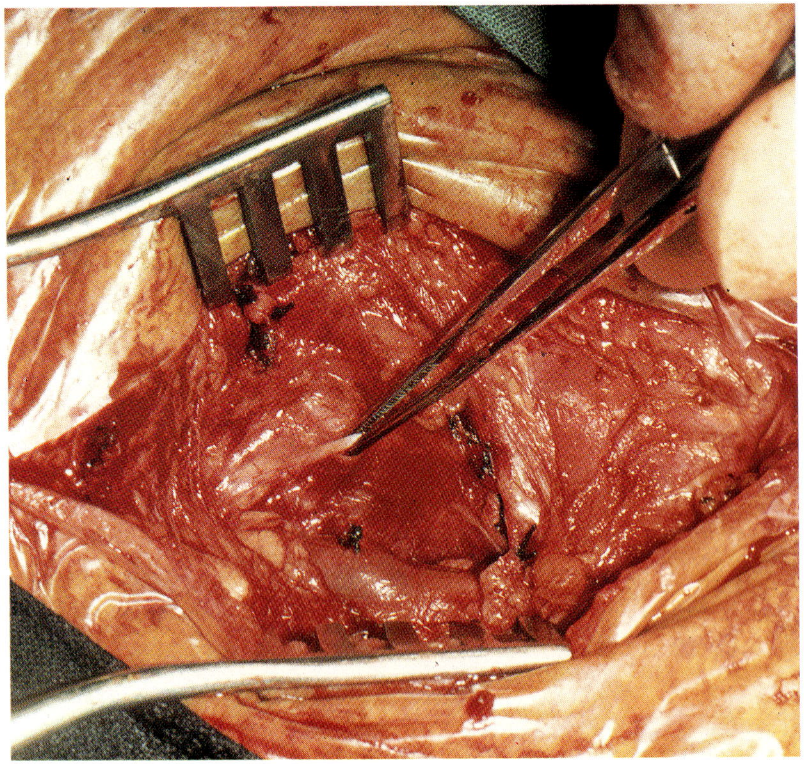

21 The descendens branch of the hypoglossal nerve is picked up (in another patient).

22

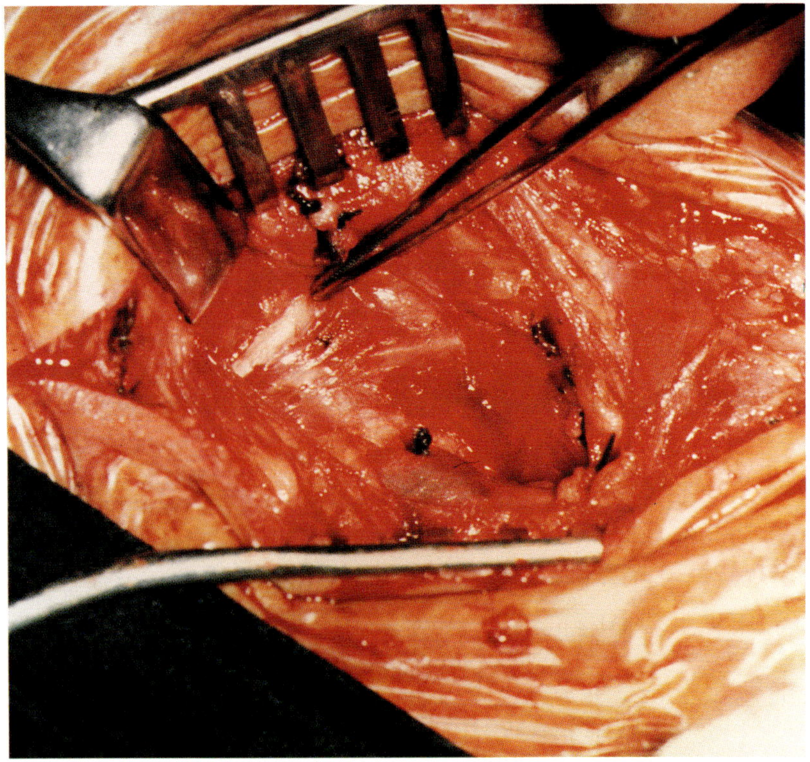

22 Traction on the divided descendens branch and upwards retraction of the wound edge reveals the trunk of the hypoglossal crossing the carotids.

23

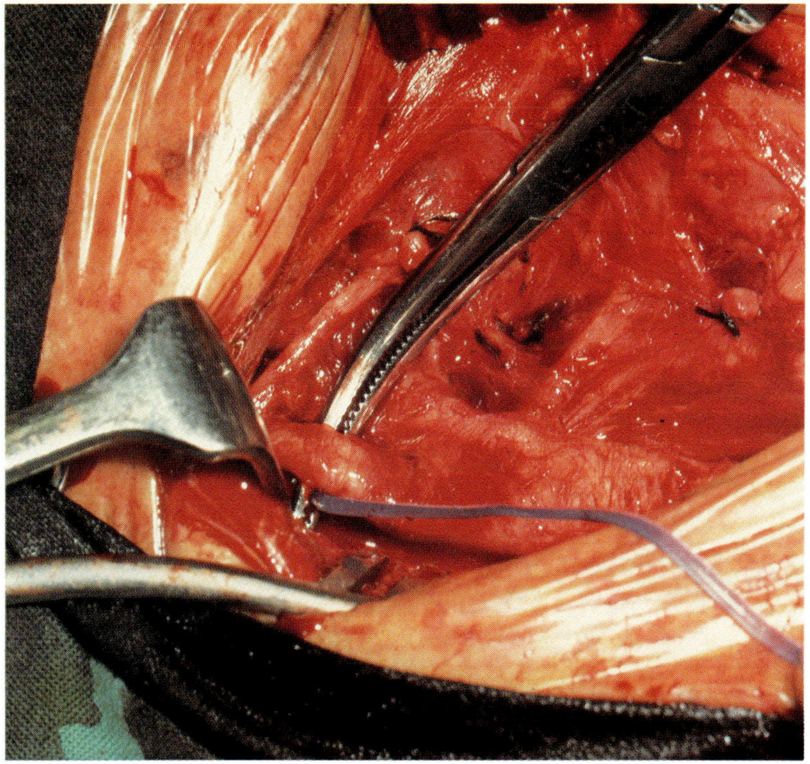

24

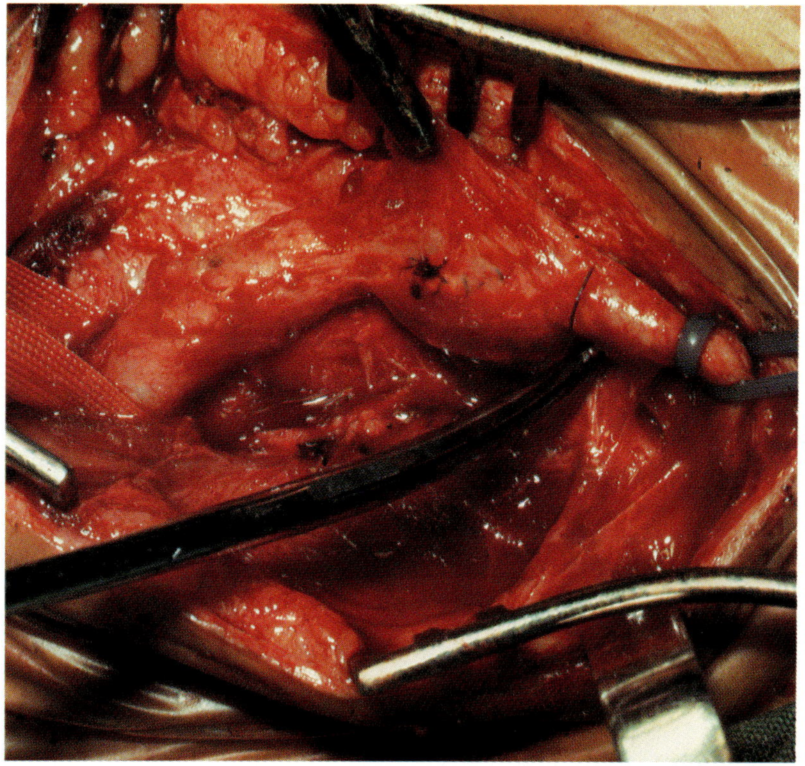

23 The hypoglossal nerve has been gently mobilised (this may require division of the sternomastoid branch of the occipital artery, around which branch the nerve may curve quite sharply when under traction). This allows the nerve to be retracted upwards to expose the upper course of the internal carotid artery in its soft, normal portion above the atheromatous segment in the carotid sinus. This safe portion of the internal carotid is then encircled with a soft fine silastic loop which is left loose.

24 The left carotid bifurcation in another patient, exposed for the third time for twice-recurrent stenosis. The internal carotid is controlled as an essential first step towards the exposure and mobilisation of the densely adherent bifurcation, manipulation of which, before clamping, could easily cause an embolic stroke. The danger area in this case is marked by the previous suture material. Repair by venous patch graft.

25

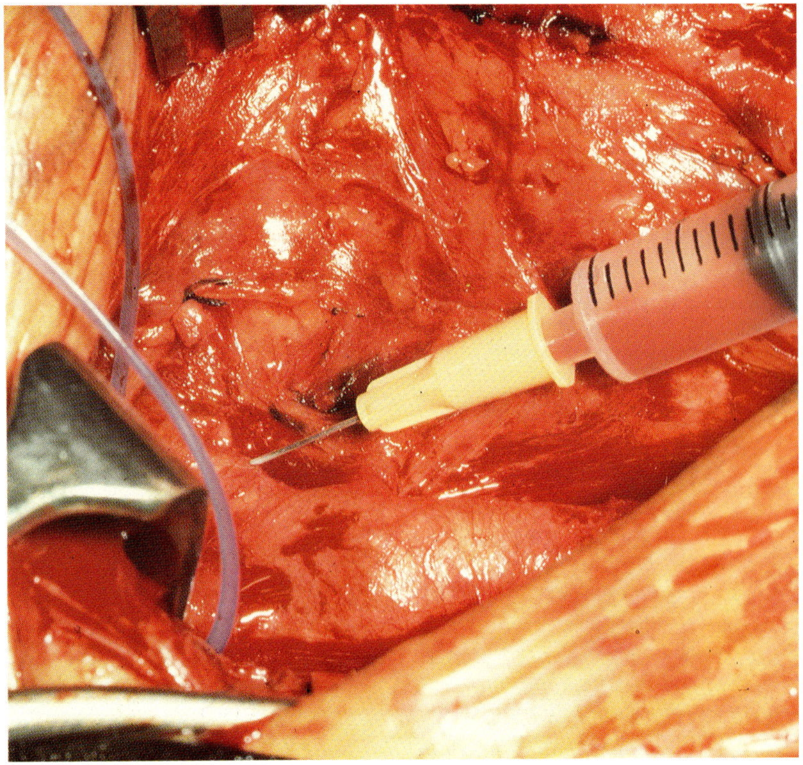

25 Heparin, 5,000 units in 1 ml is injected gently into the external carotid artery.

26

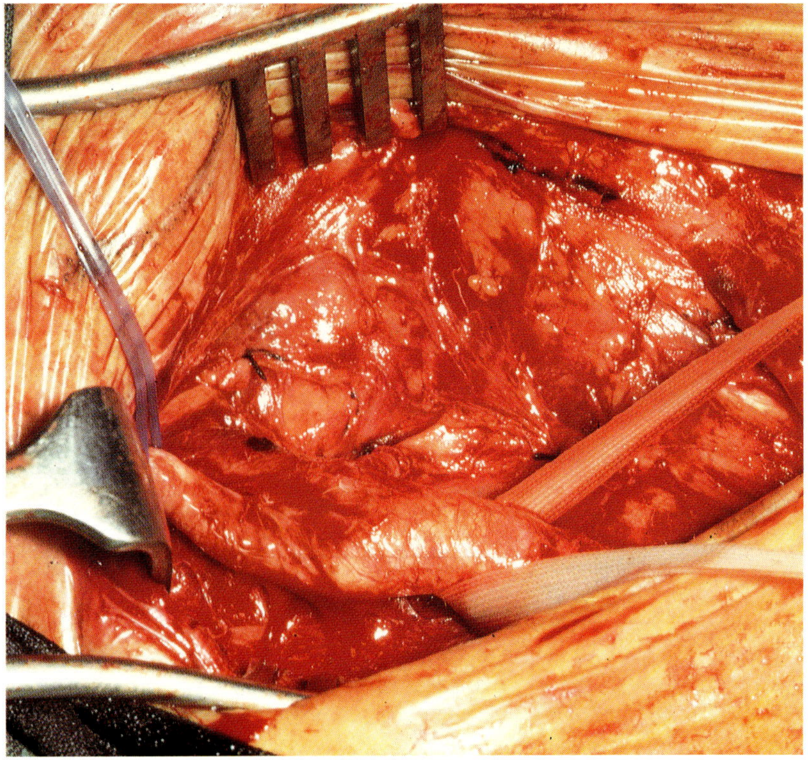

26 The silastic loop is tightened and the stopwatch recording the total carotid occlusion time is started.

27

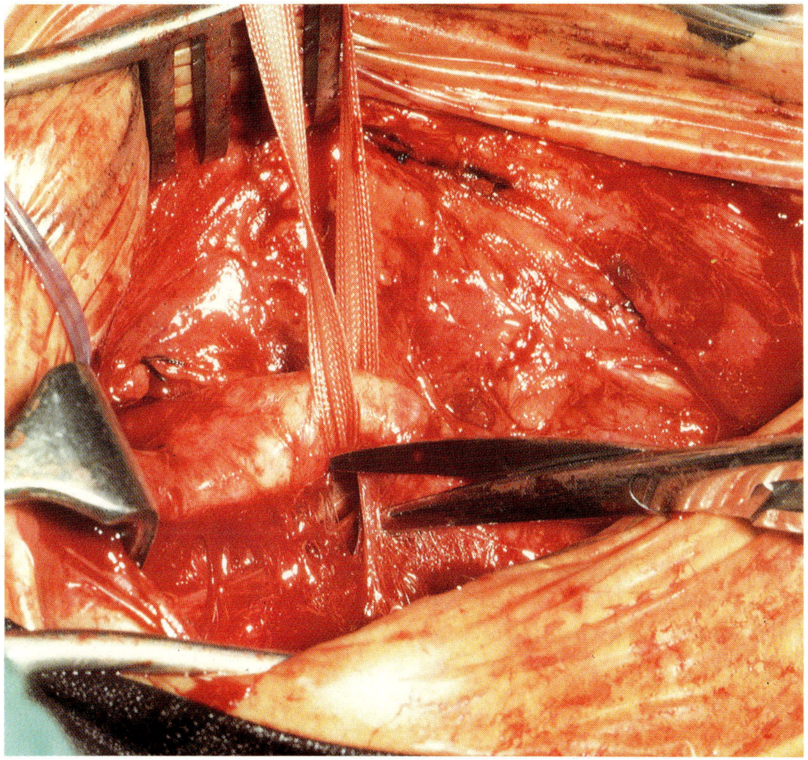

28

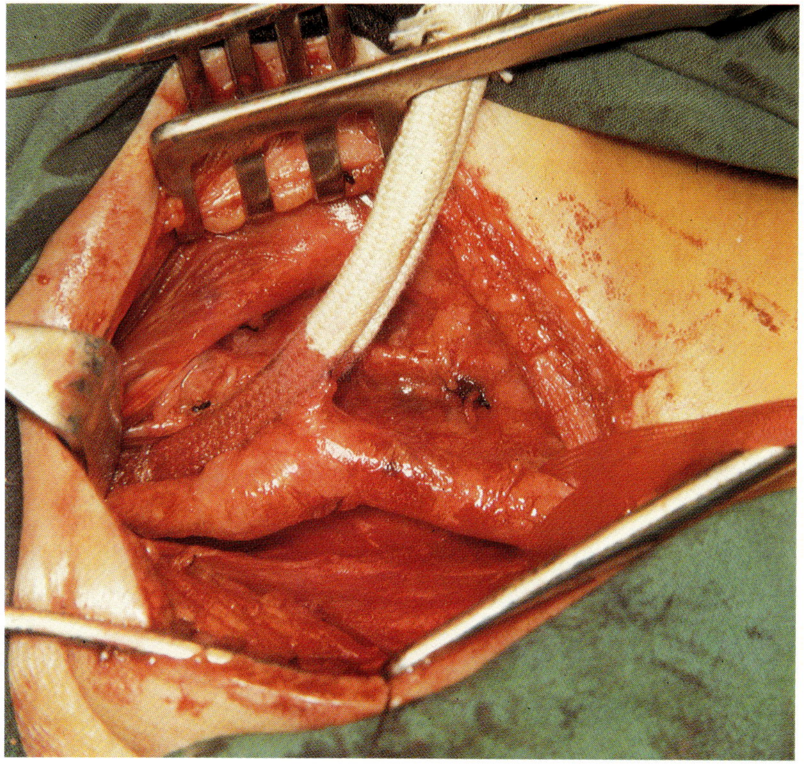

27 The common carotid and its bifurcation may now be safely and quite quickly mobilised without risk of causing an embolism. Care should be taken to identify the underlying vagus which may be adherent to the artery. Dissection between the carotids may cause hypotension or cardiac irregularity, which can be checked by the injection of xylocaine 2 per cent into the area, which blocks the afferent sinus branch of the glossopharyngeal nerve.

28 Mobilisation of the bifurcation being complete, the external, and then the common carotid are now clamped with Crafoord's cloth-covered aortic clamps. These are gentle and secure, and also serve to lift up the bifurcation into the centre of the wound. Dardik's clamps are also satisfactory.

29

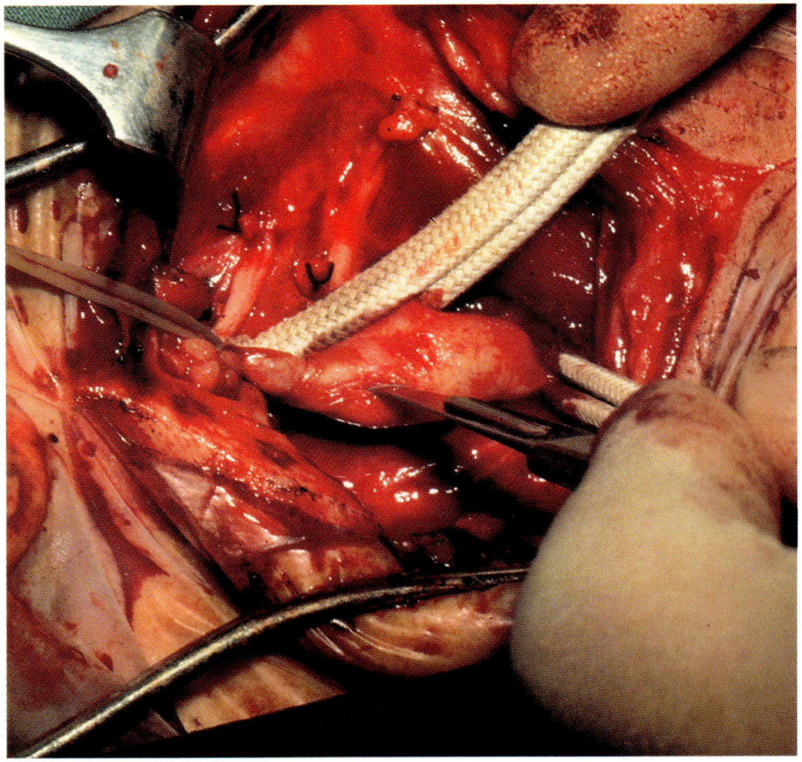

29 The initial arteriotomy is made with a No. 15 blade over the most rigid part of the carotid lesion, steadying the vessel with the external carotid clamp, or with the left index finger supporting it beneath.

30

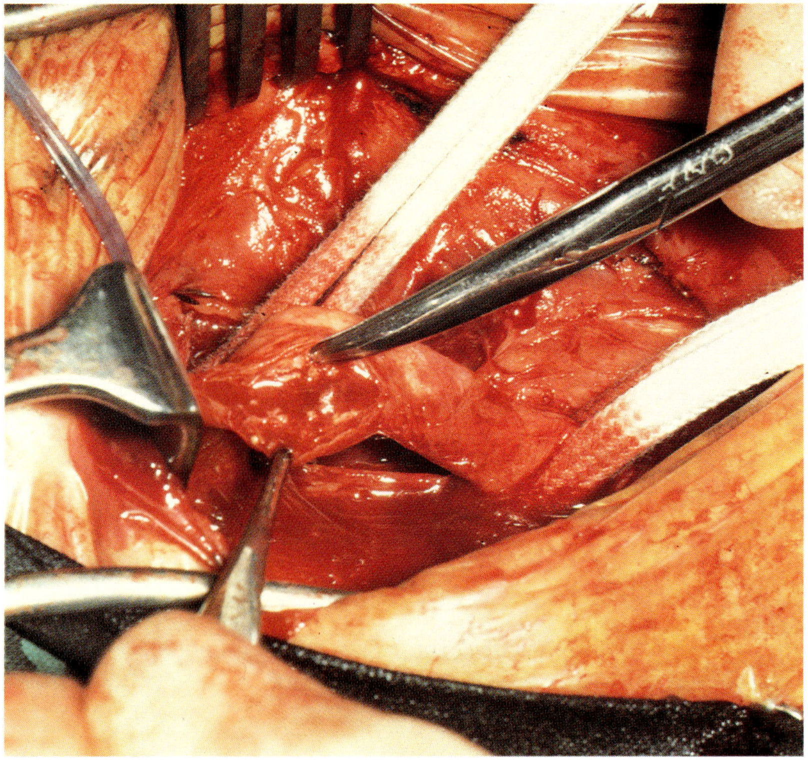

30 The arterial incision enters the lumen through the plaque layer which is irregular in consistency with crumbly, loose atheromatous material in free communication with the lumen. It is this debris that is probably responsible for the majority of perioperative strokes associated with carotid endarterectomy.

31

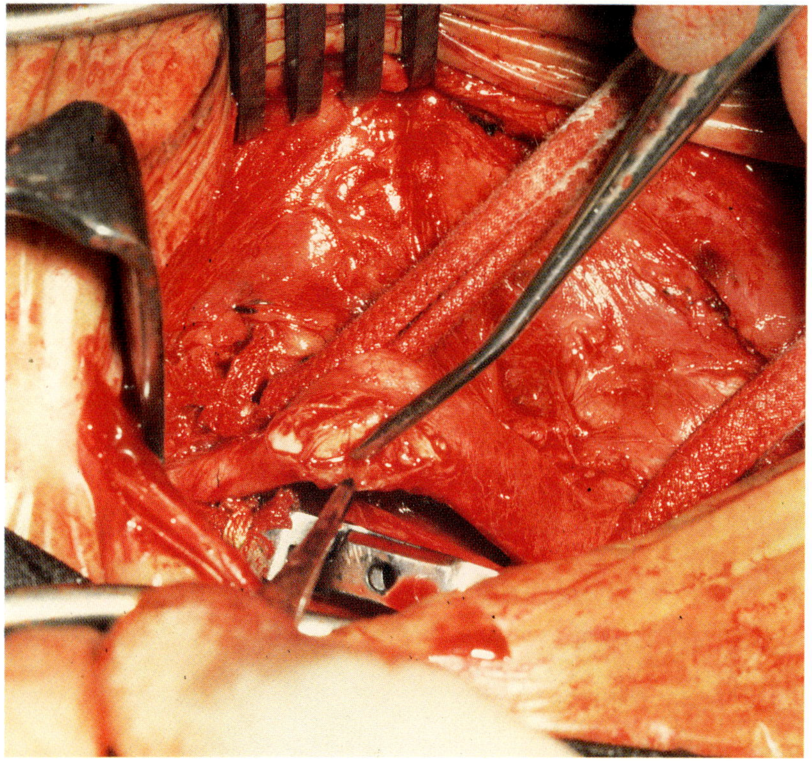

31 Having cleared and dried the arteriotomy field, the endarterectomy plane is easily found and developed at the outermost layer of the plaque, close to the adventitia, using a Watson Cheyne probed pointed dissector.

32

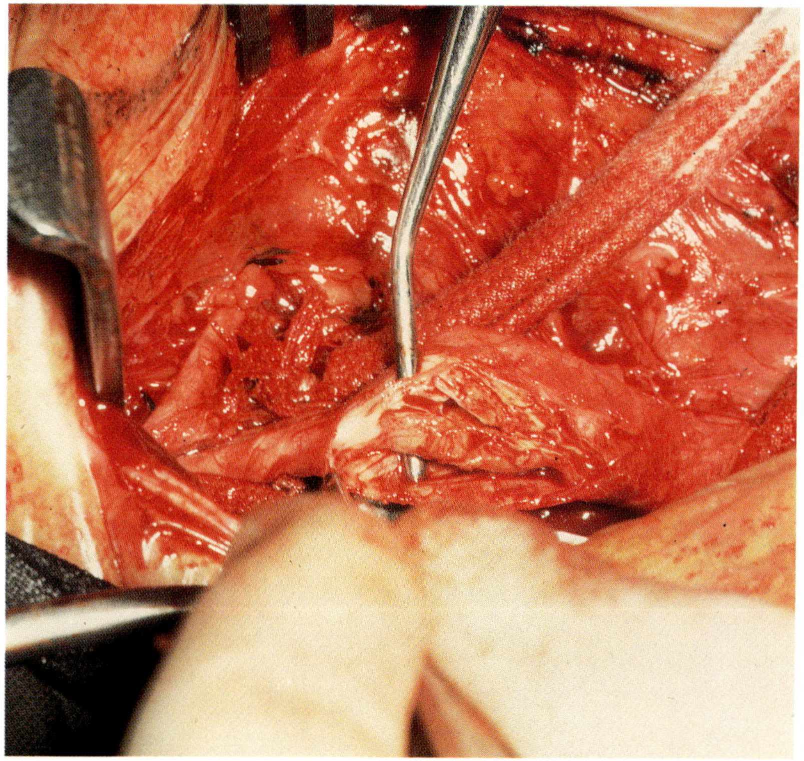

32 Taking care to remain in the same cleavage plane on all aspects of the plaque or roll of atheroma, the upper limit is carefully identified, at which level the intimal surface is smooth and normal looking, though it may be slightly raised by a tongue of atheroma, usually on the posterior aspect.

33

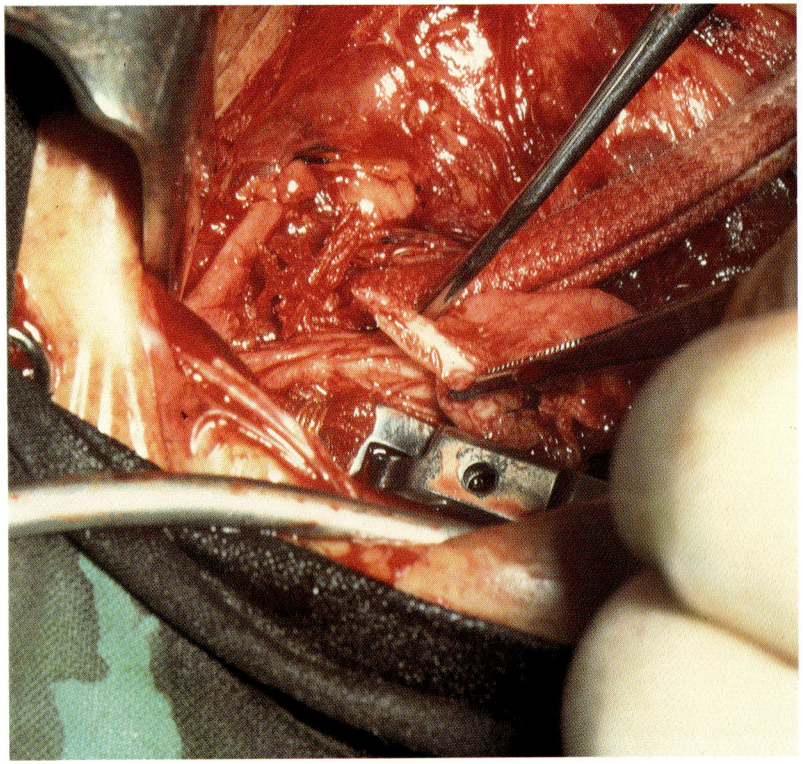

33 Often, as in this case, there is a tapering tongue of atheroma that lifts cleanly out of the upper end of the arteriotomy. . . .

34

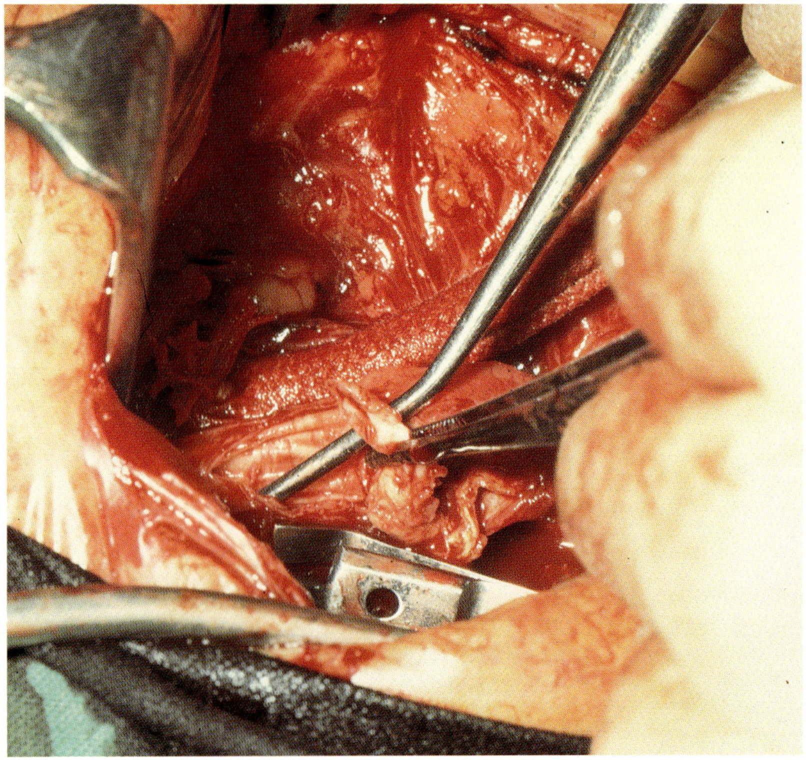

34 . . . leaving a fine, stable intimal layer at the point of separation. Securing stitches to the distal margin are seldom needed in this operation. (This appears to be a feature of the stenotic atheromatous lesion in arteries of high resting flow, in contrast to the femoro-popliteal, for example, in which plaque morphology is laminar and extensive).

35

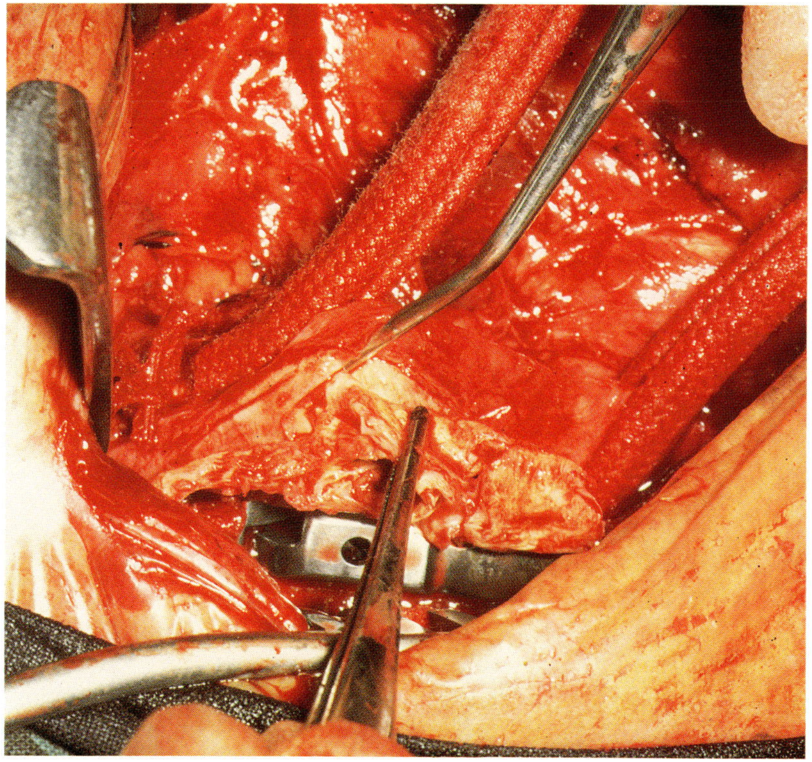

35 Entering the endarterectomy plane into the external carotid. The nearby Crafoord's clamp should be moved further up the artery to allow the plane of dissection to reach the branches if possible, where the distal prolongations of the main plaque can be more easily and cleanly separated with the probe, and with gentle downwards traction on the main plug, using a Dunhill's artery forceps placed well up on the atheroma in the trunk of the external carotid.

36

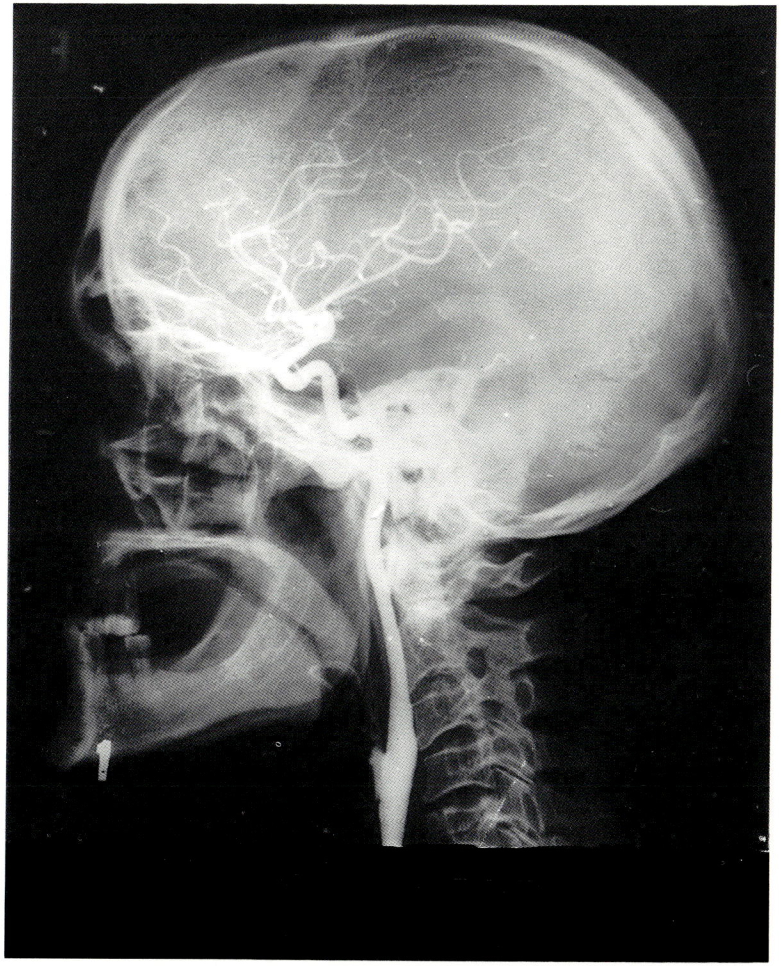

36 Postoperative arteriography often shows a deficiency of the endarterectomy as far as the external carotid is concerned.

37

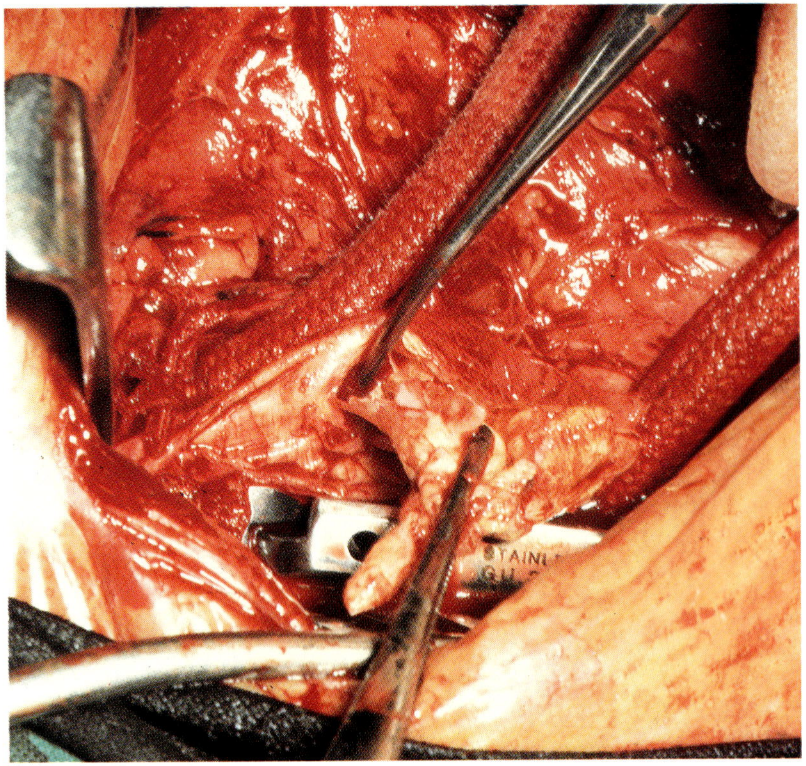

37 Finding the plane in the common carotid below the external carotid orifice.

38

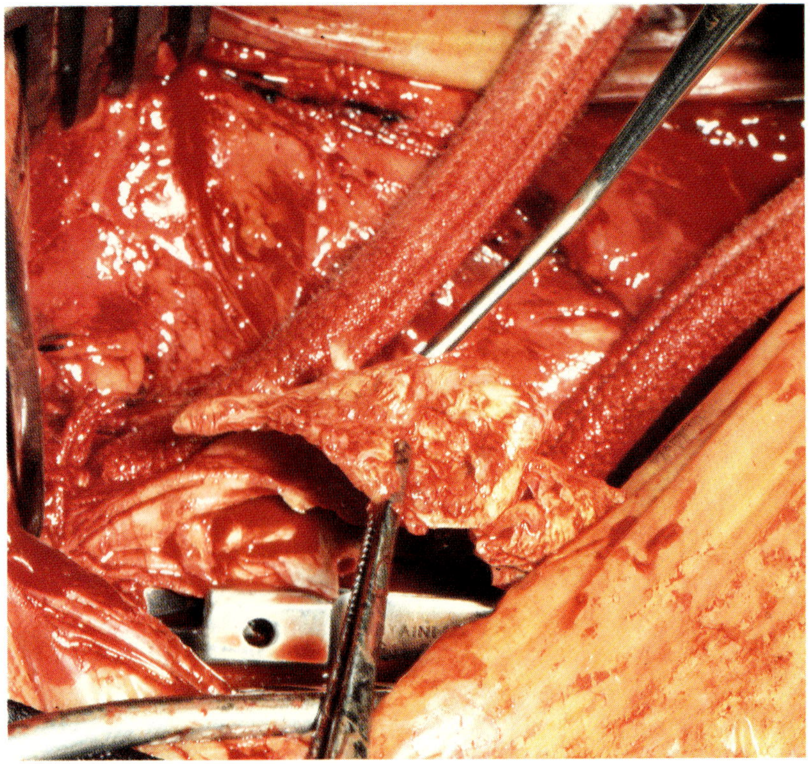

38 Endarterectomy is complete as far as the common carotid clamp.

39

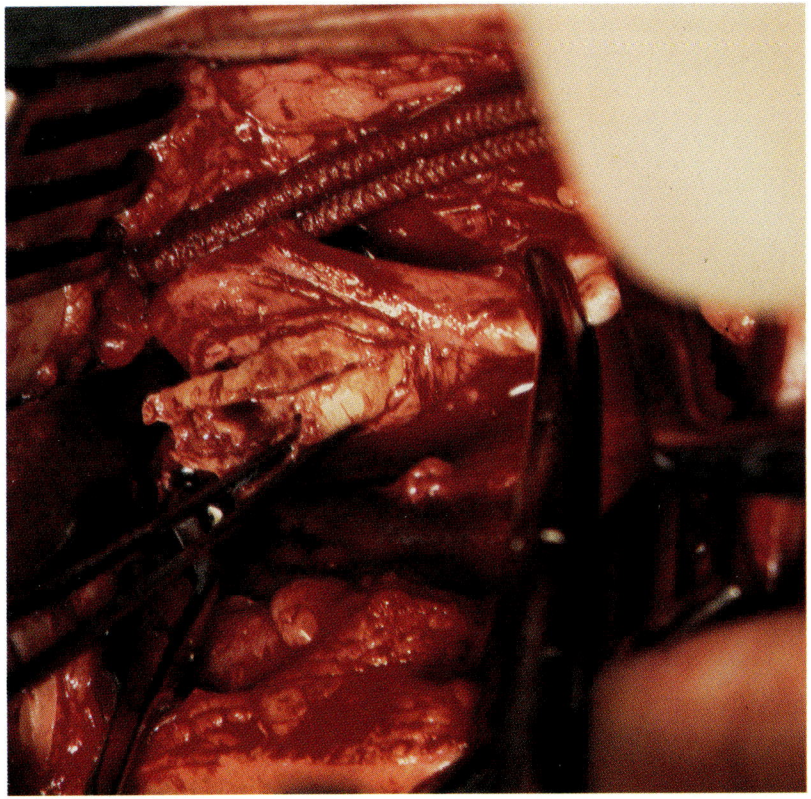

39 It may be sufficient to nip the atheroma across near this point by applying a pair of Dunhill's forceps firmly just above the clamp, when the plug will separate cleanly in many cases. If this method is used it is essential to inspect the line of division within the carotid closely for remnants that might embolise.

40

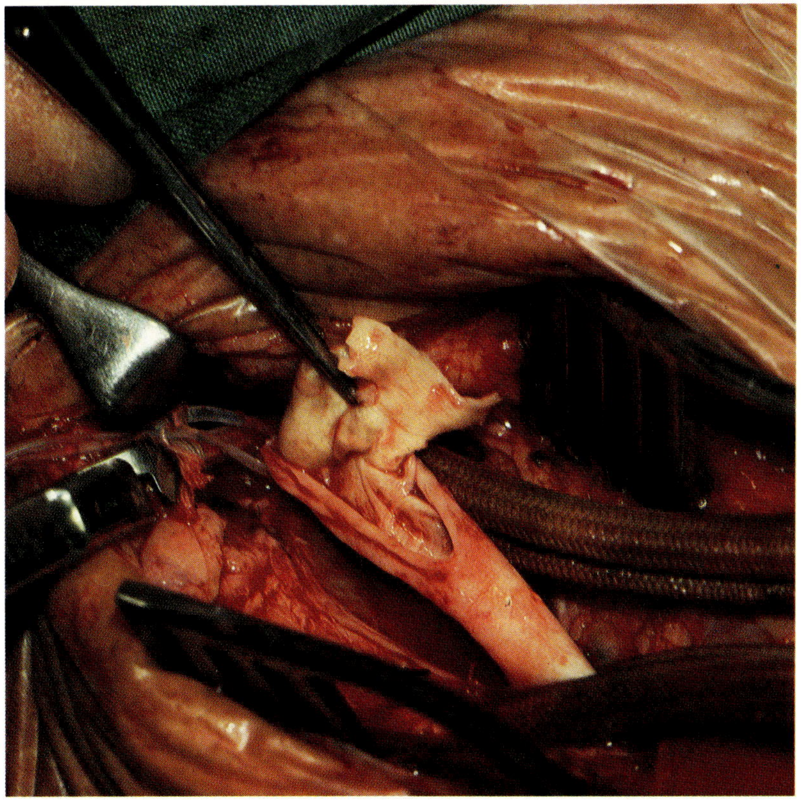

40 Alternatively, if there is adequate room, the common carotid clamp can be moved down the artery to allow of a sharp division of the plaque under direct vision (another right-sided case is shown to illustrate this point).

41

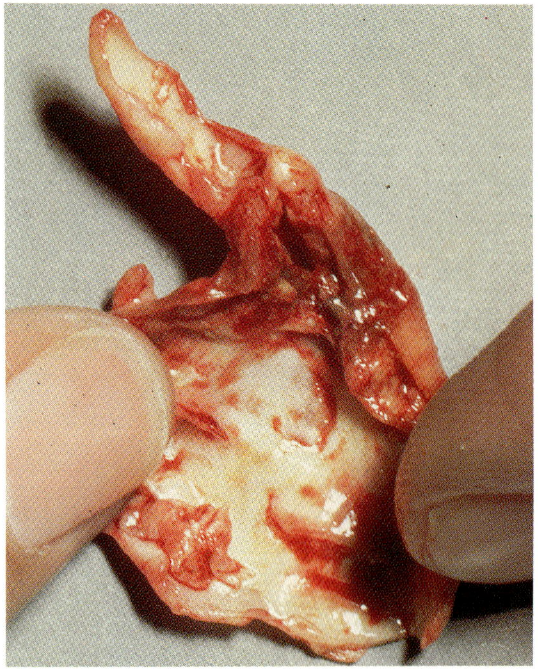

41 The separated specimen from a similar case to that shown in Figures **29** to **40**. Note the opening into a cavity that was found to be filled with soupy material.

42

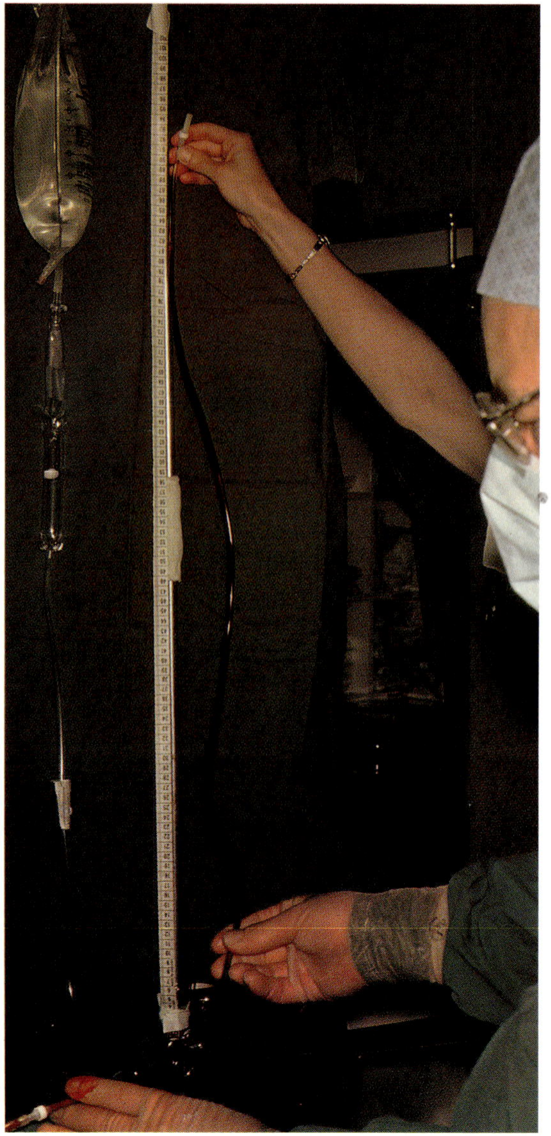

43

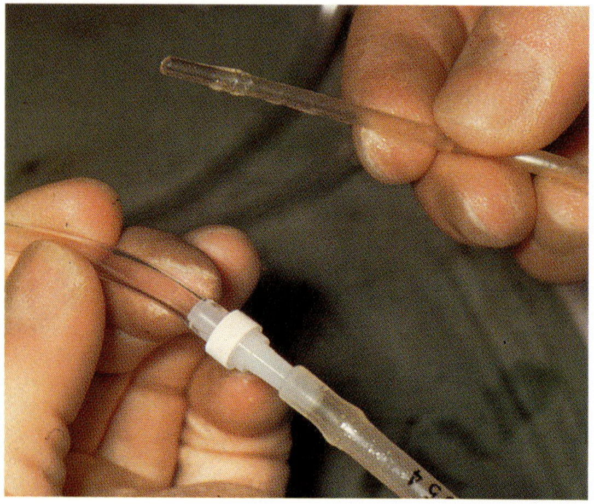

42 & 43 Measurement of internal carotid stump pressure by the author's simplified method. The larger end of a Javid's carotid shunt will be found to fit perfectly to the male end of a standard Luer gauge intravenous drip infusion extension. The distal end of the shunt is inserted gently into the cleaned and flushed opening of the internal carotid within the arteriotomy and the tubing is held vertically up against a simple measuring scale. The manometer thus constructed will fill quickly with blood in most cases and this proof of the adequacy of cerebral backflow is then measured in centimetres of blood, a scale which is a little less than ten times the value in mm Hg. Levels between 50 and 150 cm or more are considered satisfactory, the zero being placed at heart level.

44

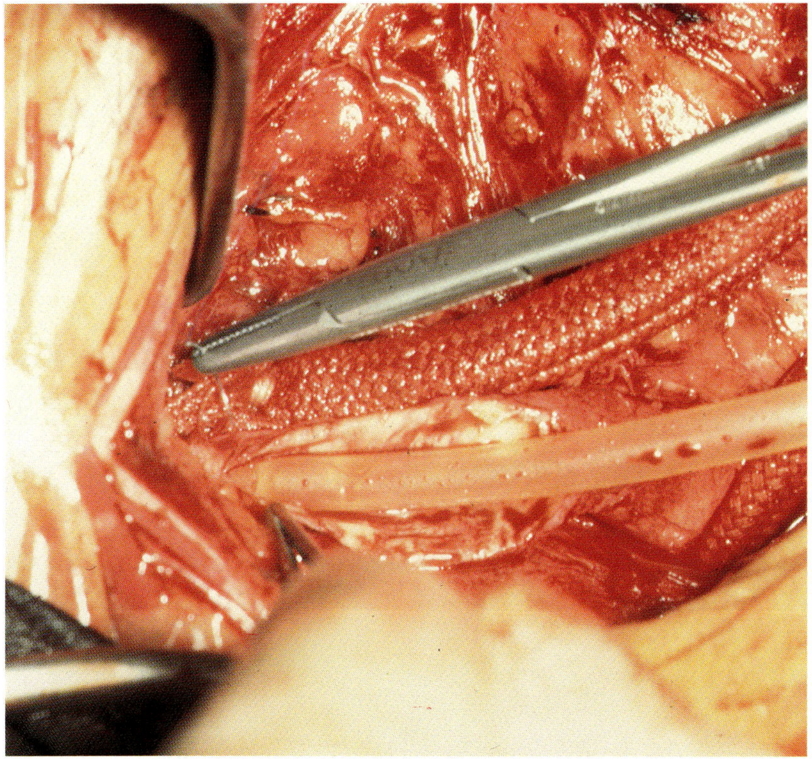

44 The same shunt can be used as a stent to assist in the correct placing of the first, important and often technically difficult distal arteriotomy closure. Continuous 6/0 polypropylene is used.

45

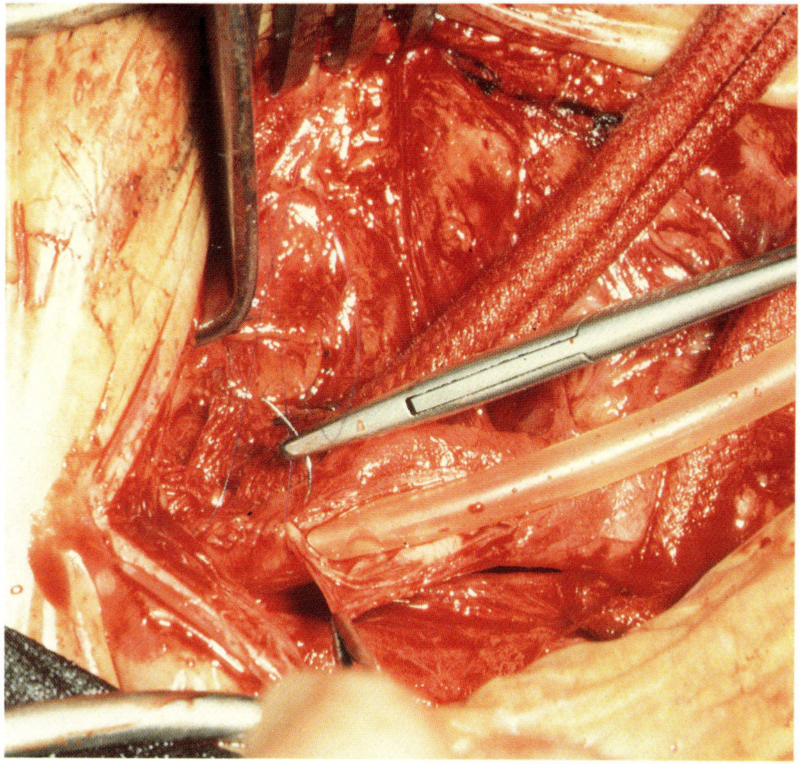

45 The distal first centimetre of the arteriotomy has been closed, and the wider lumen of the sinus is reached. The shunt can now be removed from the internal carotid and a bulldog clip or Dardik clamp is placed just above the top suture.

46

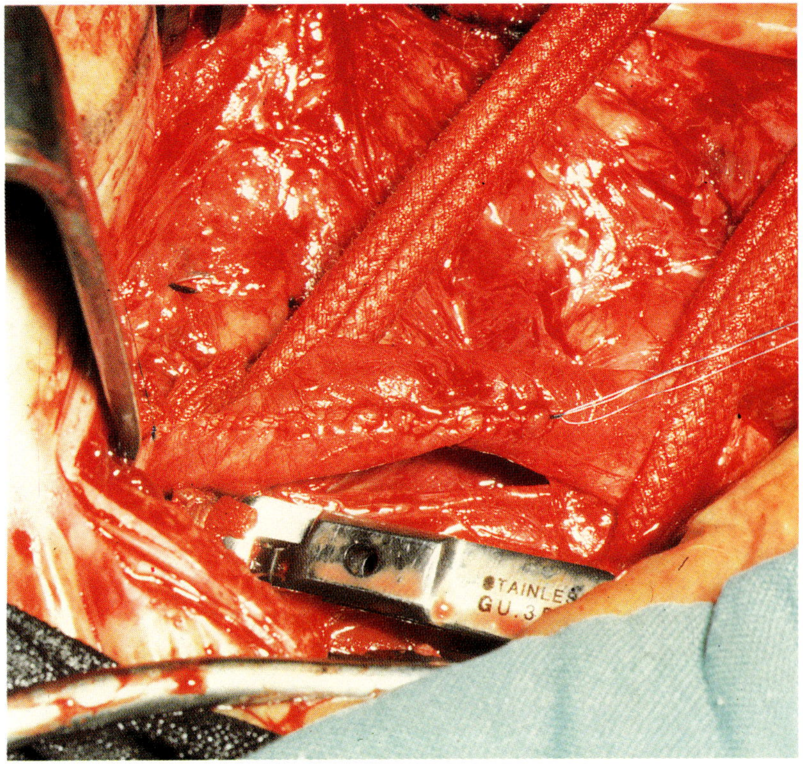

46 Arteriotomy repair is complete, all three clamps are still in place, heparin has not yet been reversed.

The indwelling carotid shunt

A full insertion of the Javid shunt may be required under the following circumstances:

1. Carotid stump pressure below 50 cm blood (40 mm Hg).
2. A residual neurological defect.
3. Opposite carotid occluded or severely stenosed.
4. Technical difficulty anticipated (e.g. a long or high plaque, or if a vein patch is needed for recurrent stenosis).

The shunt is flushed and filled from above and its lower end is gently inserted into the common carotid, which is held a little lower down with the finger and thumb to control the lumen while the shunt is passed down between the fingers. A Javid ring clamp is then secured over the neck of the slight bulb at the tip. The same method will have been used to fix the upper end of the shunt in the internal carotid.

47

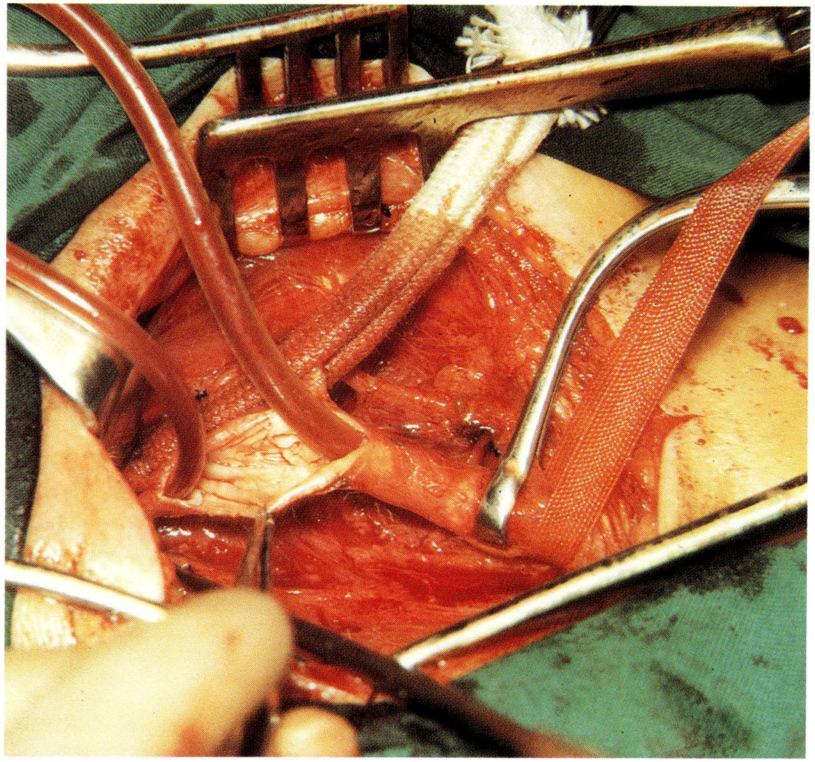

48

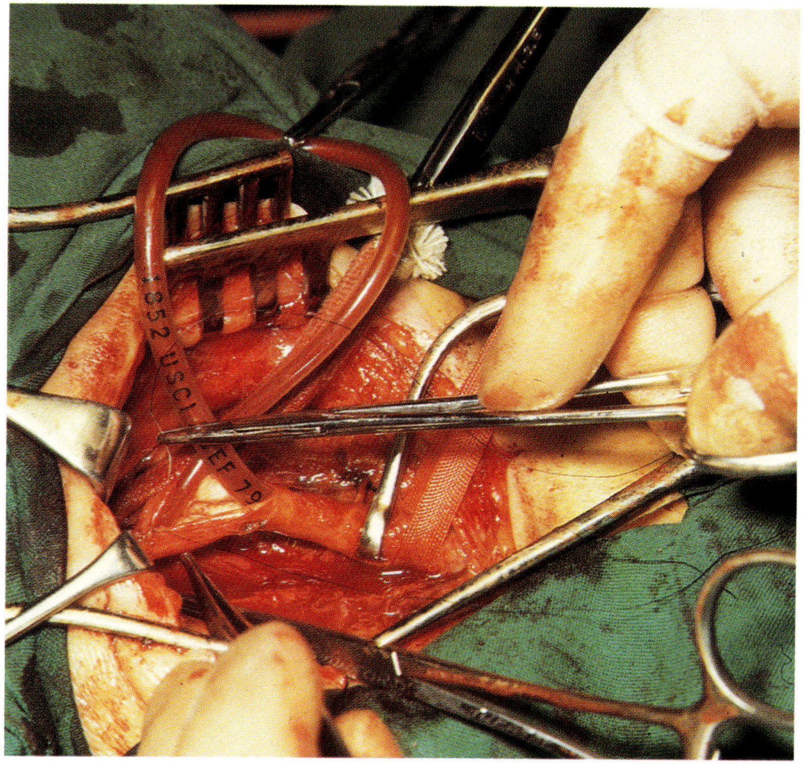

47 Shunt in place, opened out and held aside to show the completeness of the endarterectomy and to allow for final detailed cleaning of any loose remnants. Most surgeons have found difficulty in performing the endarterectomy with the shunt in place, particularly at the ends of the plaque, and will complete it before inserting the shunt. The time taken for this is quite short in comparison with the repair phase, which is the real purpose of the shunt.

48 The shunt is looped and held forwards to allow more room for the suturing of the arteriotomy. The artery forceps seen at the apex of the looped shunt is not applied, but is resting on the tubing.

49

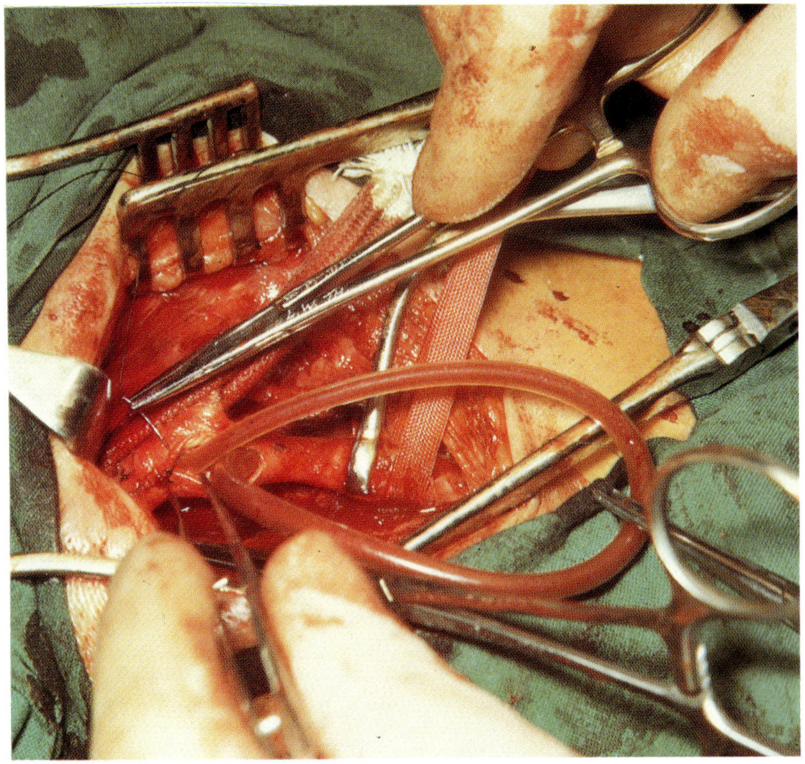

49 Drawing the shunt downwards allows as many as possible of the last few sutures to be inserted with the shunt still in place. The opened lumen is flushed with heparin saline before closure.

50

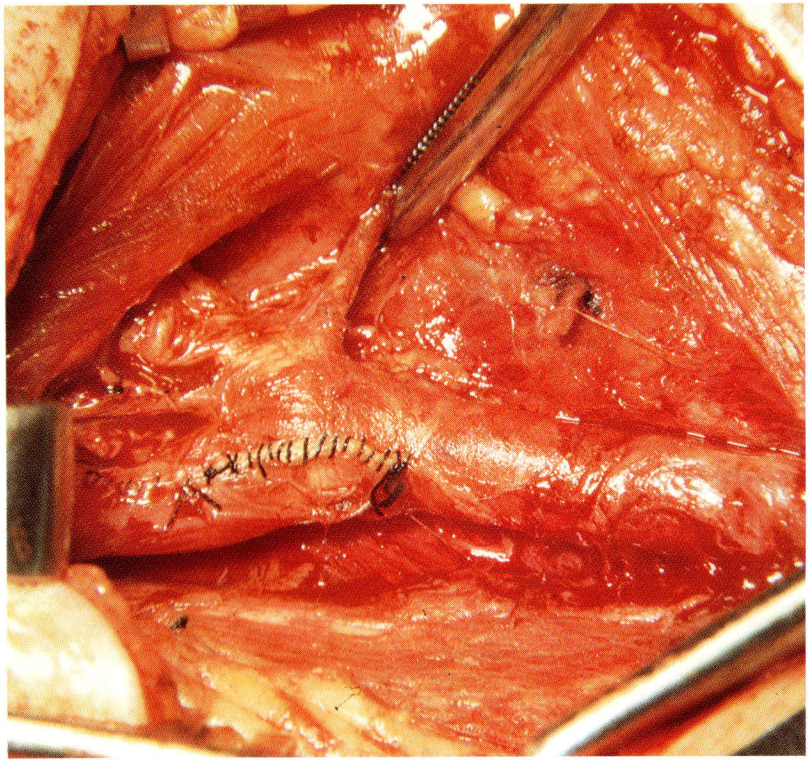

50 Completed arteriotomy closure. For the lower wider and more thicker walled portion it is worth using a slightly heavier suture, such as 5/0 polypropylene or braided polyester. This will hasten the conclusion of the repair, and is often more suitable than 6/0.

51

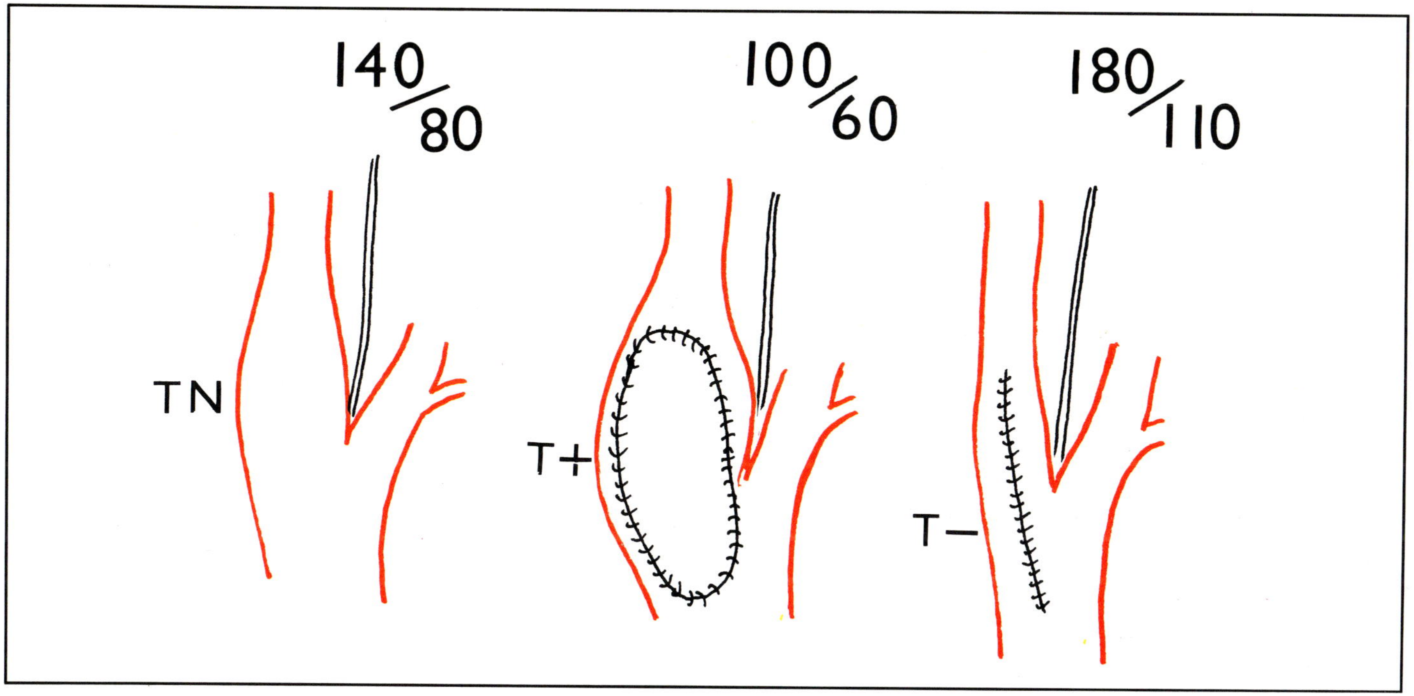

51 The effect of post-repair carotid sinus diameter upon blood pressure regulation through the sinus branch of the glossopharyngeal nerve. (TN = wall tension normal, T + = wall tension increased, T − = wall tension reduced.)

Order of clamp removal

52
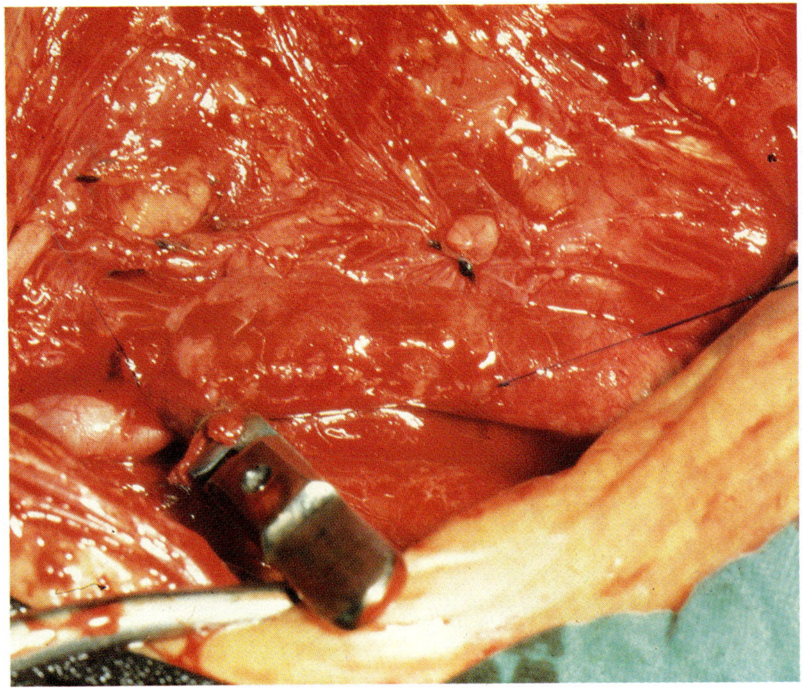

53
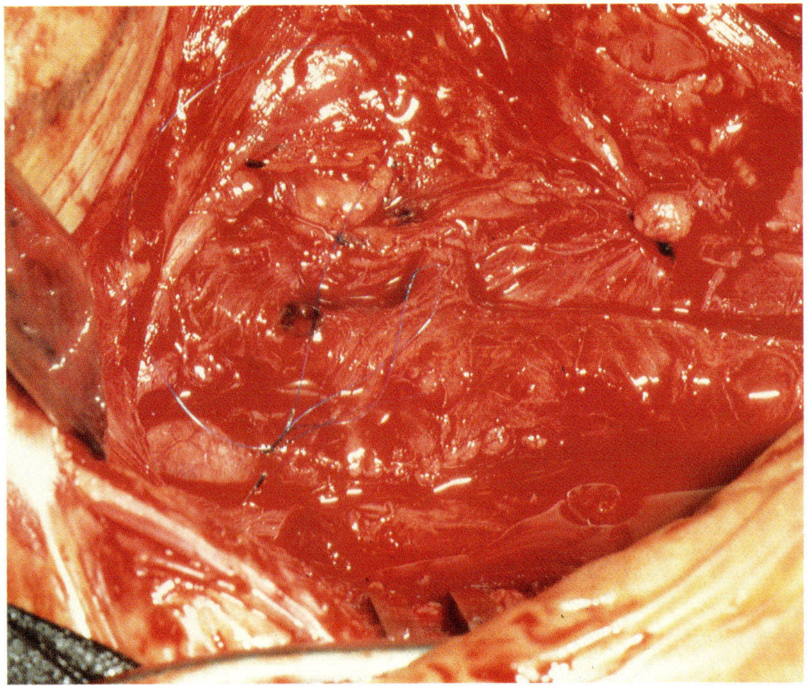

52 The bulldog clamp on the internal carotid has been moved down to the bifurcation, close to the origin of the external carotid, which tests the haemostasis of the upper suture line. The common carotid clamp is now taken off, then the external carotid, which proves the security of the main repair, and the patency of the external carotid. It also ensures that any unnoticed loose material that might still be present in the lumen is carried safely into the external distribution and not into the brain.

53 All clamps removed; stopwatch clamp time recorded; moderate oozing from still-heparinised repair.

54

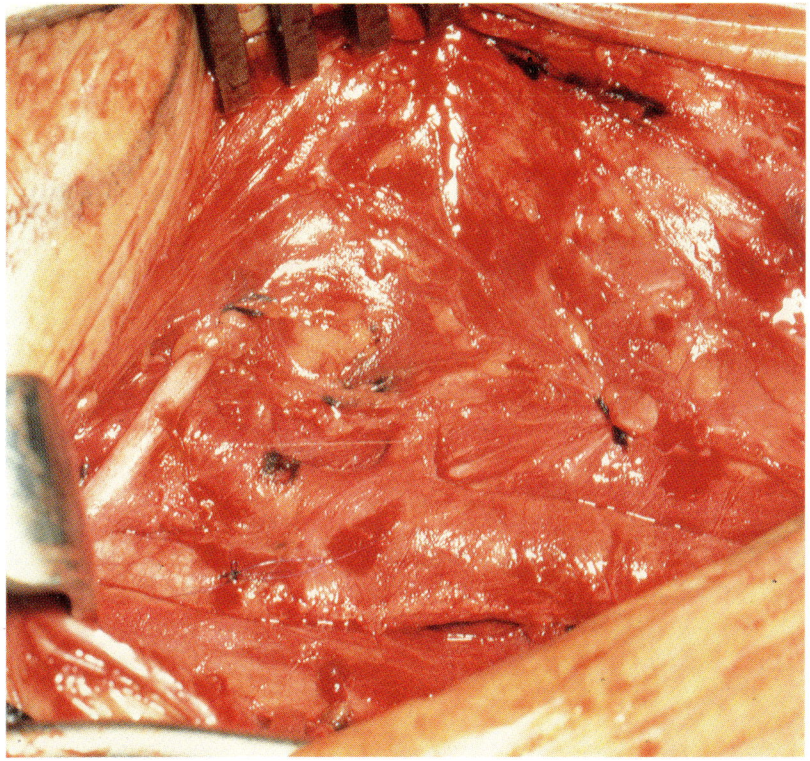

54 A few minutes after the intravenous administration of 100 mg protamine sulphate by the anaesthetist the field has ceased to ooze.

55

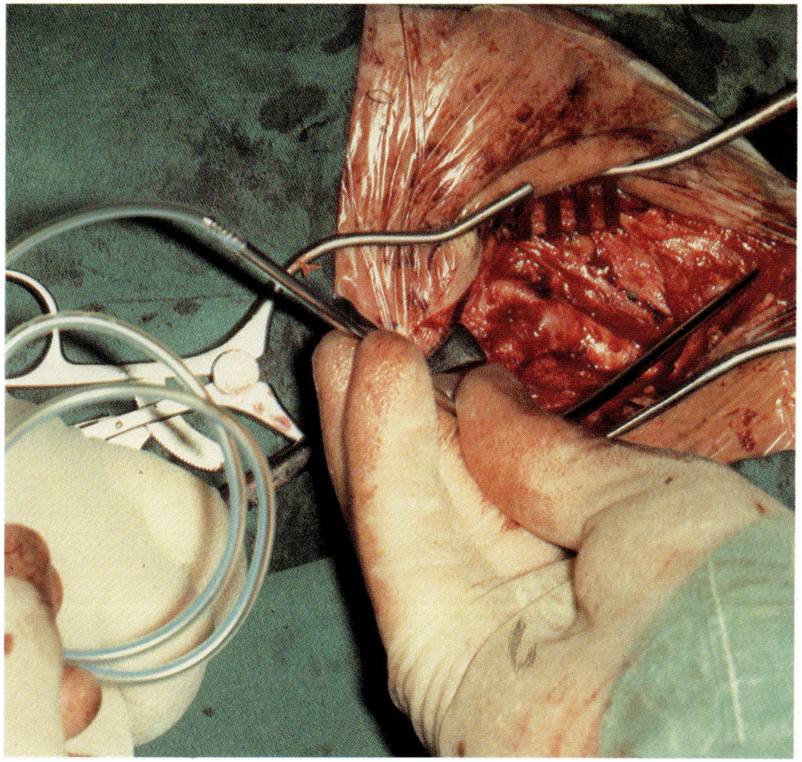

55 A vacuum drain is passed with its trocar through the lower end of the wound.

56

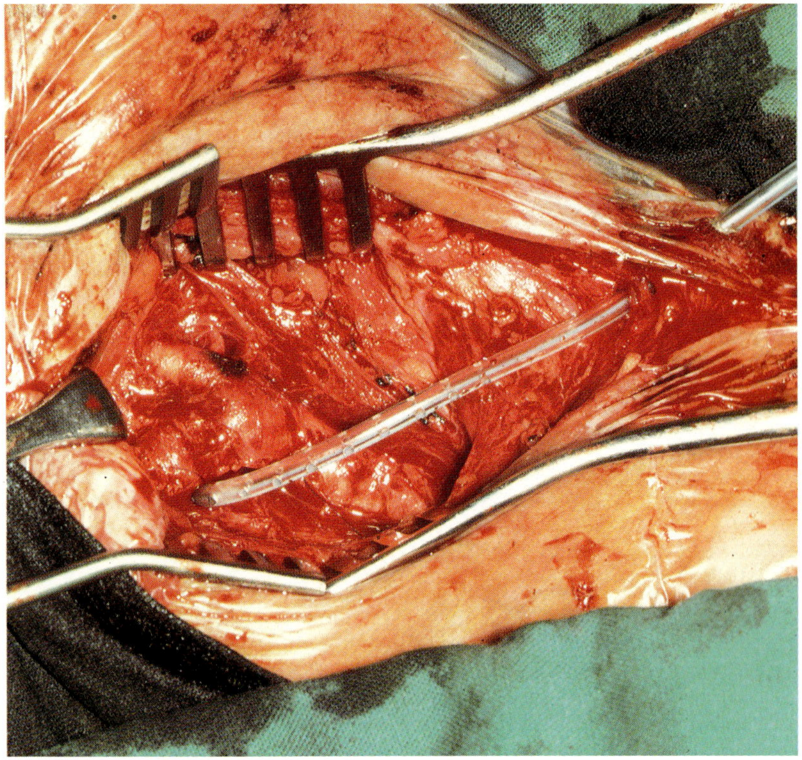

57

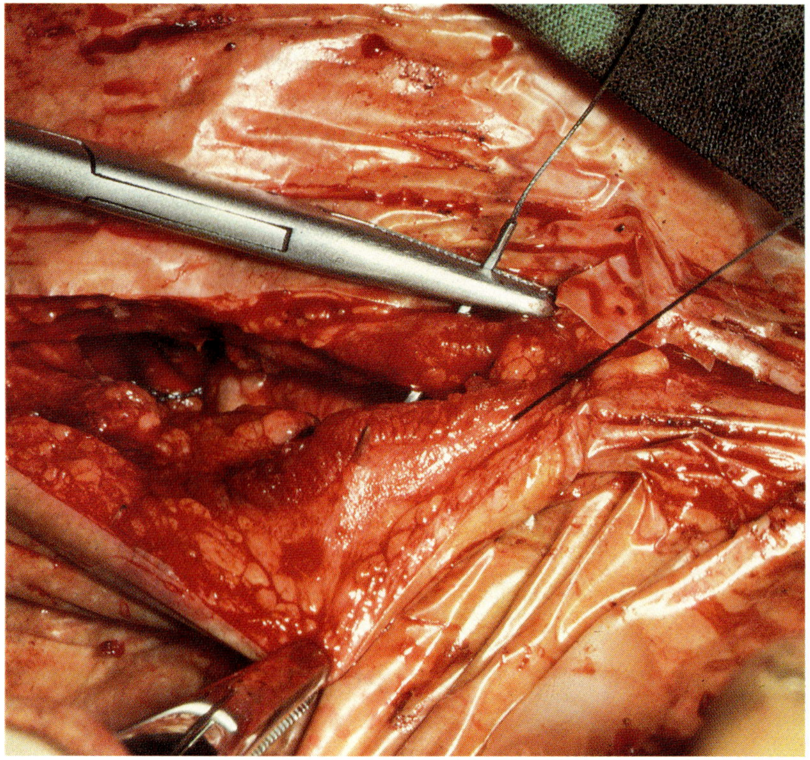

56 The tip of the drain is cut across so as to lie loosely over the carotids.

57 Deep fascial closure with interrupted 2/0 polyglycollic sutures. Continuous sutures might lead to compression effects within the wound on the vessels or the airway in the event of postoperative bleeding.

58

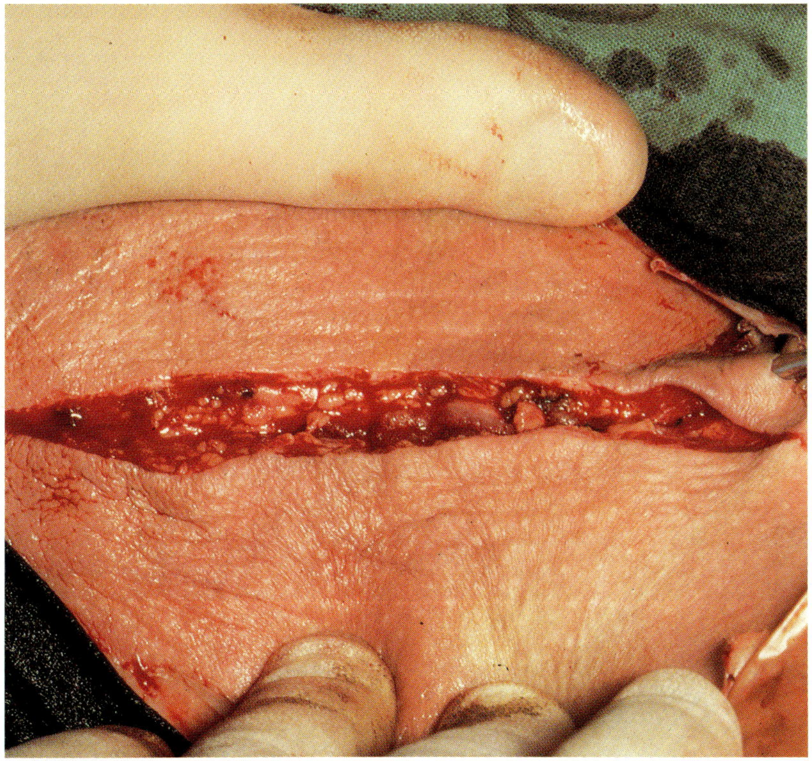

58 Interrupted subcutaneous sutures of the same material with ends cut close to the knot.

59

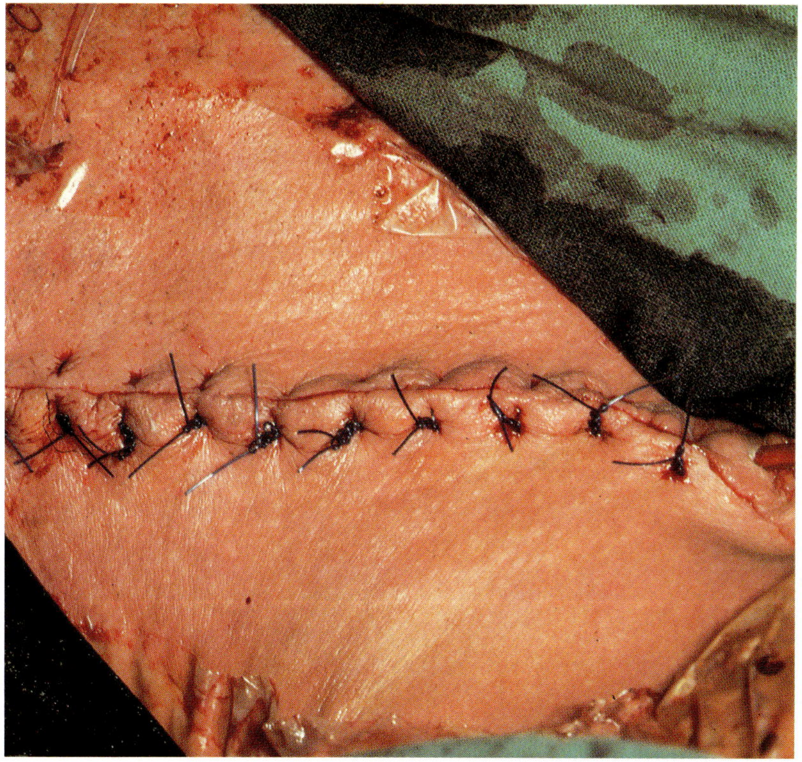

59 Skin closure with interrupted 3/0 nylon. Silk securing stitch around the point of emergence of the vacuum drain.

Postoperative care

Close supervision is essential during the first 12 to 24 hours, in a well staffed recovery or intensive care area. Quarter-hourly blood-pressure monitoring is maintained, and a careful observation is made of the neurological signs, with regard to limb movement and level of consciousness. Stroke may still occur, though the patient may have awakened neurologically intact. Technical failure from early occlusion of the repair may be commoner than is believed, for it need not cause neurological damage. An immediate or early-developing defect should raise the question of immediate re-exploration, particularly if the blood pressure has been steady. Non-invasive testing, e.g. of the supraorbital blood velocity with the Doppler may help this decision. Where available digital intravenous subtraction angiography should be carried out.

One of the commonest features of impending early postoperative stroke is the development of hypertension. Any pre-existing infarct may thus become haemorrhagic. Minor lesions, not clinically apparent before operation may be tragically revealed in this way. Should therefore the blood pressure begin to rise significantly during recovery, e.g. from a steady 150/80 to 180/95 or more a hypotensive drug should be given. Hydralazine 10 mg into the intravenous infusion will control the milder cases, but sodium nitroprusside must be ready in case it does not. 50 mg in 500 ml dextrose saline is set up, and the drip rate closely and continually regulated to bring the blood pressure down to its previously normal level.

Almost as dangerous is a fall in blood pressure; this requires volume replacement with dextran. This complication is less common if the sinus nerve has been divided. Most patients return to normal ward care on the first morning after operation. Thereafter recovery is rapid and smooth, though careful vigilance is still necessary for 3 or 4 days in case of the development of other cardiovascular complications. The commonest of these is a myocardial infarct.

The average patient leaves hospital on the fifth postoperative day, and may return to normal activities in 2 or 3 weeks.

Cranial nerve defects are commoner than is realised: hypoglossal weakness 5 per cent, hoarseness from vagal retraction or temporary cord weakness on routine laryngoscopy 25 per cent, sensory disturbances of the skin area near the wound 60 per cent; most of these are minor disabilities and almost all resolve spontaneously.

Mortality from this operation should not exceed 2 per cent and the incidence of *new strokes* should be less than 5 per cent. Late strokes should not exceed 10 per cent, though as we have seen recurrent stenosis or occlusion may occur without ill effect in as many as 20 per cent.

Carotid body tumour

The operative treatment of these uncommon tumours is made difficult by their extremely close and vascular adherence to the carotid bifurcation. Most cases are symptomless, usually affecting young or mature women in their most active years.

With a major risk of hemiplegia if the carotids have to be ligated for control of operative haemorrhage most surgeons therefore feel a reluctance to operate, particularly as the tumour is slow growing and seldom metastasises. Yet, the longer operation is delayed the worse the local problem becomes, with increasing arterial involvement and the tumour tending to envelop important nearby structures such as the hypoglossal nerve. Often the neck has already been explored. This, especially if some attempt has already been made to mobilise or resect the tumour will greatly magnify all the technical difficulties.

Indications for surgery

In general, simply the presence of the tumour. The case for resection is strengthened when the lump is confined to the region of the angle of the jaw, and if it retains slight lateral mobility on the main vessels.

60

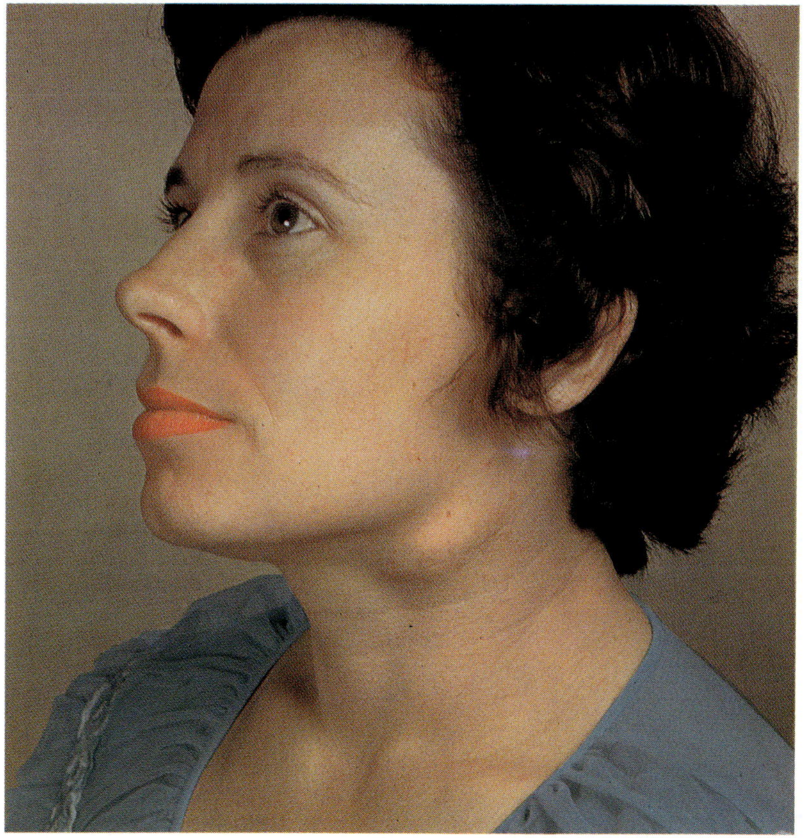

60 In this typical patient a limited biopsy exploration had already been done, the oblique scar from which can be seen. A soft arteriovenous murmur was present, as in perhaps 25 per cent of cases.

61

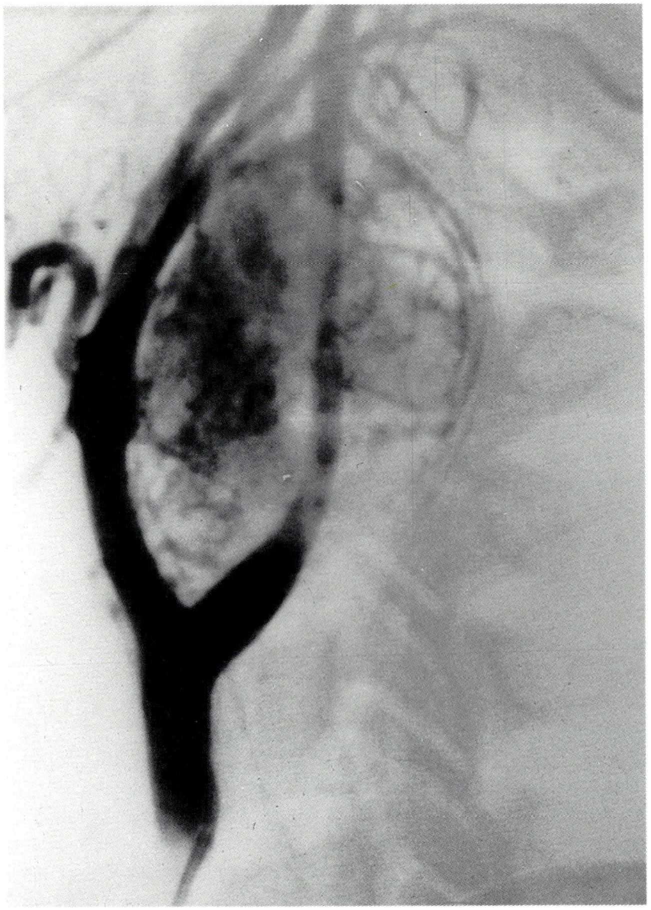

61 Arteriography in the case shown in Figure **60** confirms the diagnosis ("goblet" widening of the intercarotid space with rich vascular filling) also the limited extent of the tumour (rounded upper outline, with few abnormal vessels outside the main mass).

Contraindications

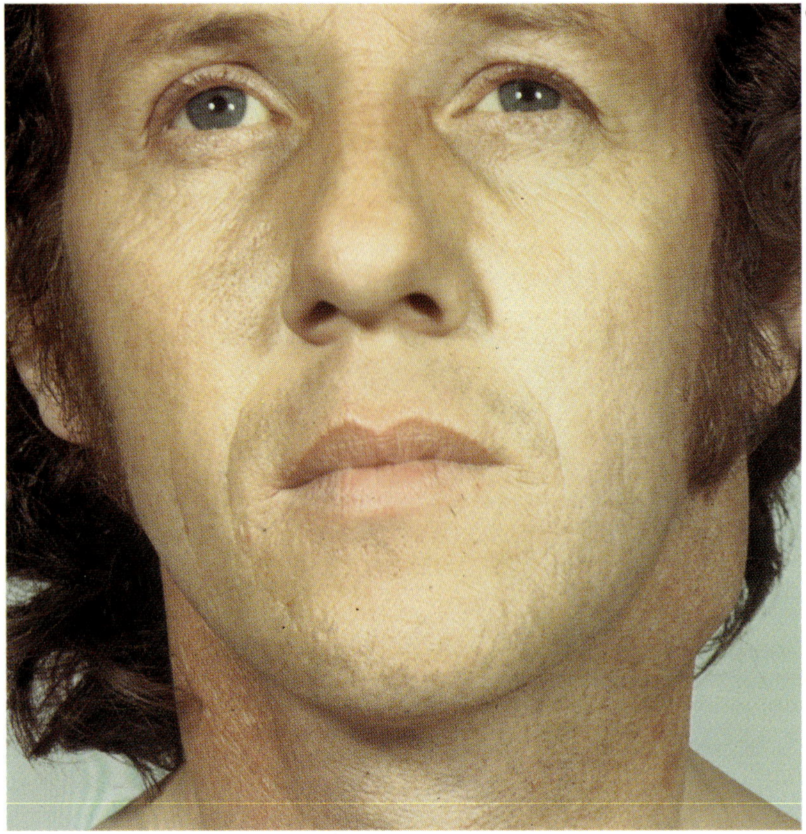

62

62 An inoperable case. Although on clinical examination this tumour appeared to be limited to the region of the carotid bifurcation at operation the lesion proved to be extensive and highly vascular, with no clear line of separation. Biopsy however confirmed that it was a chemodectoma.

63

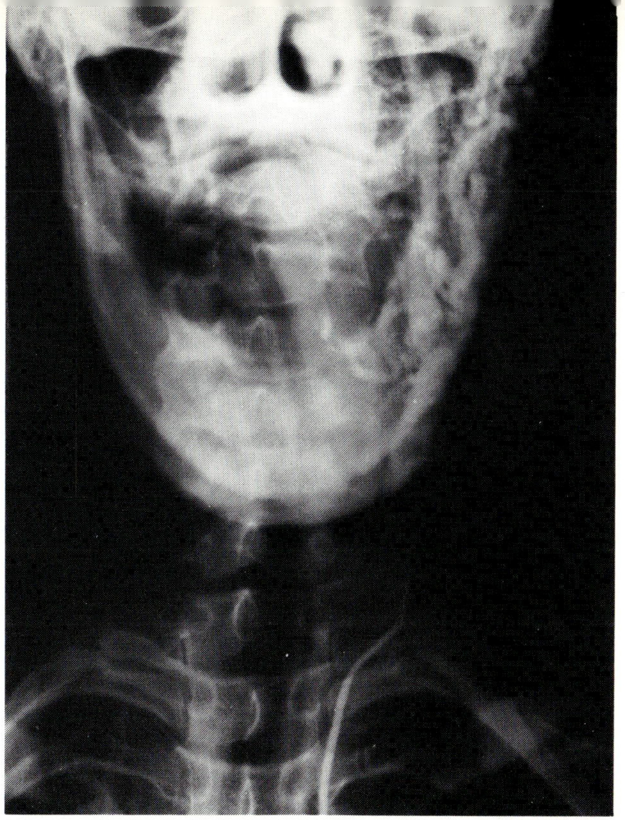

65

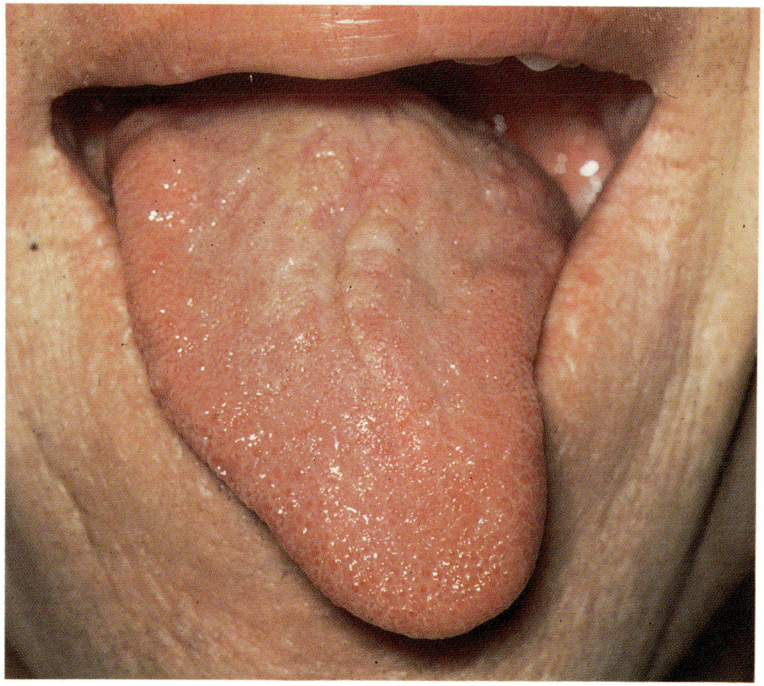

64

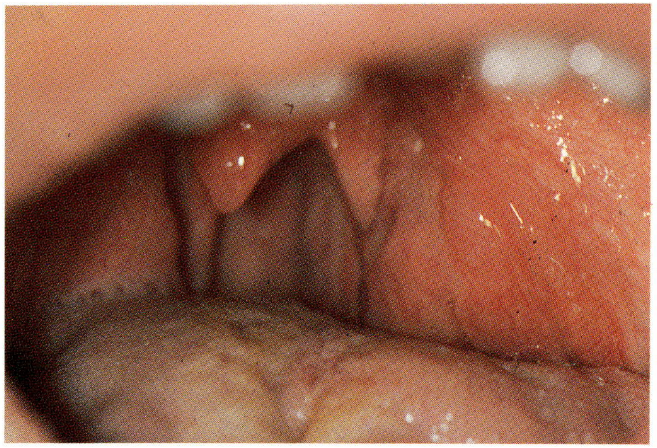

63 The arteriogram in this case contrasts with that shown in Figure **61,** confirming the widespread and infiltrating nature of the tumour with no clear outline or limit.

64 Preoperative clinical examination had shown that tumour was present above and behind the soft palate.

65 There was already hemiatrophy of the affected side of the tongue, owing to hypoglossal nerve involvement. He had also been noticed to have a left sided Horner's syndrome (Figure **62**).

Treatment of suspected inoperability

Exploration and biopsy should be advised, but the patient should be spared the risk of mutilation and disability that attempted radical excision can cause. Radiotherapy can be effective in controlling or reducing the tumour. The patient shown in Figure **62** remains well after 11 years. The remnant of the lesion, just below the mastoid process measures 1 cm.

Excision of a carotid body tumour

66

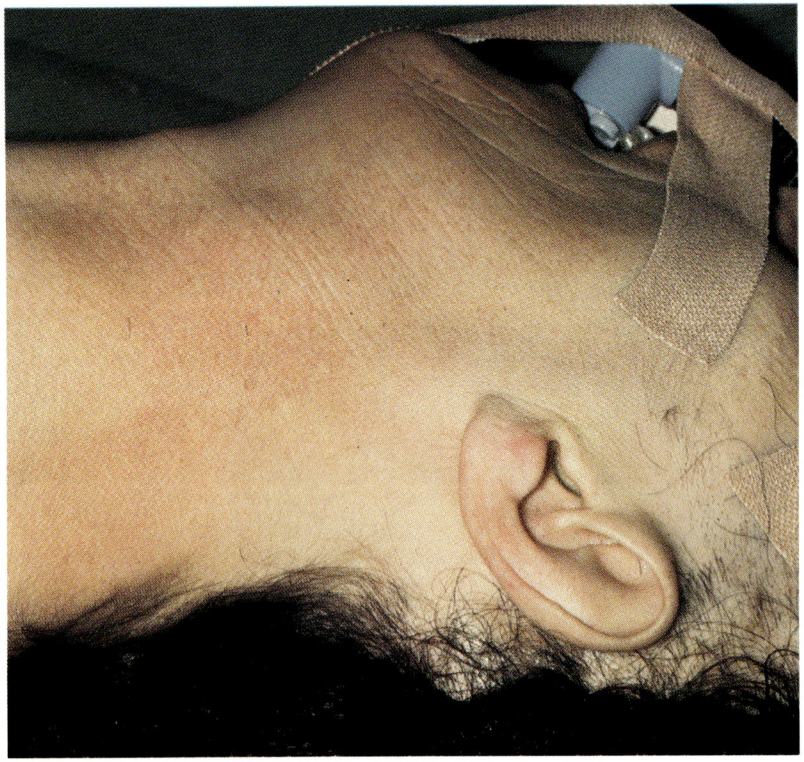

66 The patient is positioned with the neck well extended, with the tumour presenting well at the centre of the field.

67

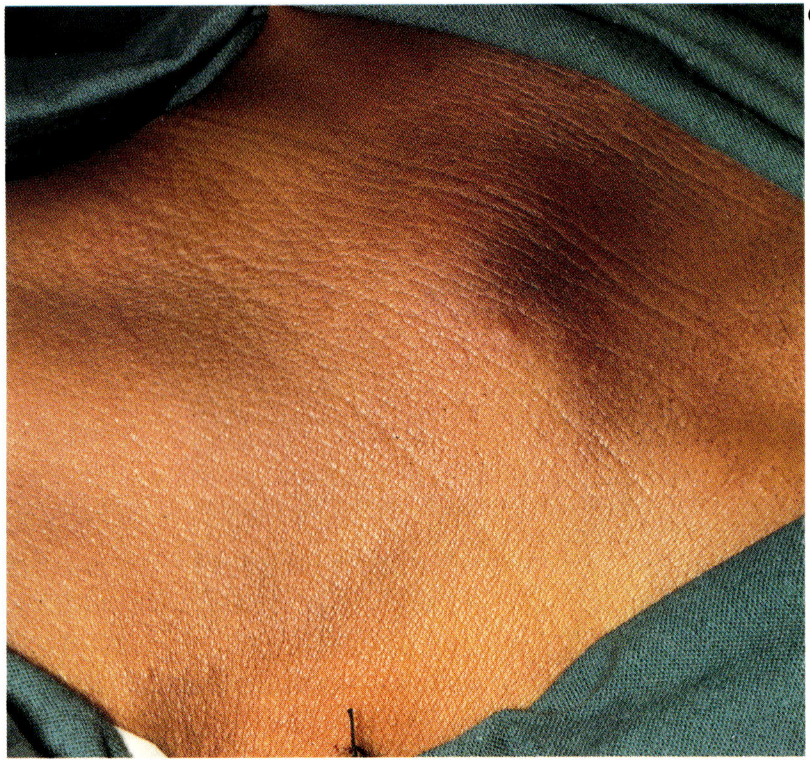

67 The skin drapes are applied. (See also Figure **10**.) The incision is the same as for carotid endarterectomy.

68

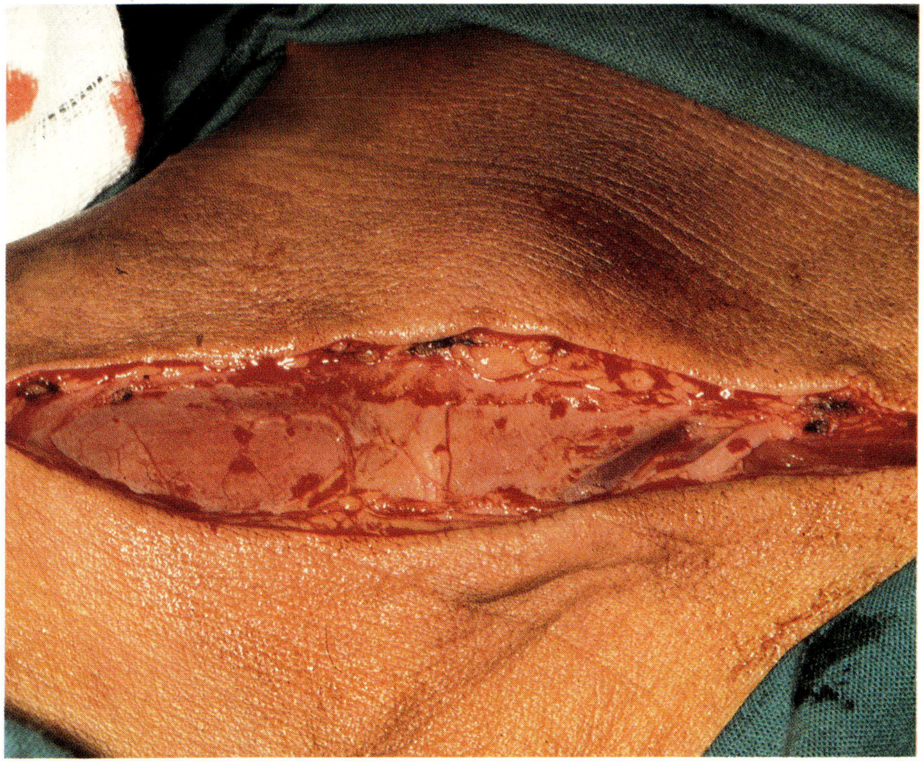

68 Exposure of the deep fascia; cutaneous nerves cross at the centre and upper parts of the incision (transverse cutaneous and great auricular; the latter should be separated and preserved).

69

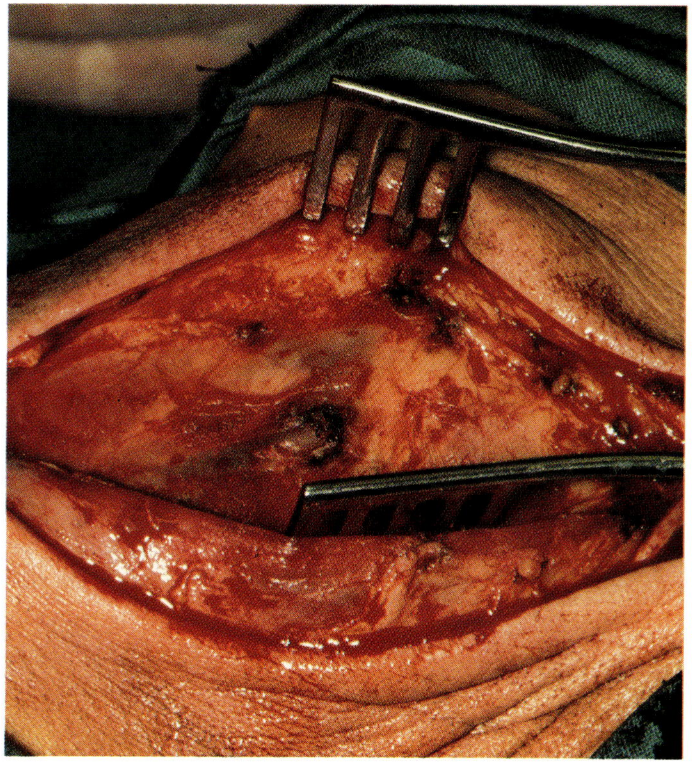

69 The deep fascia incised along the anterior border of the sternomastoid muscle. Travers' self-retaining retractor is inserted in a preliminary, shallow position.

70

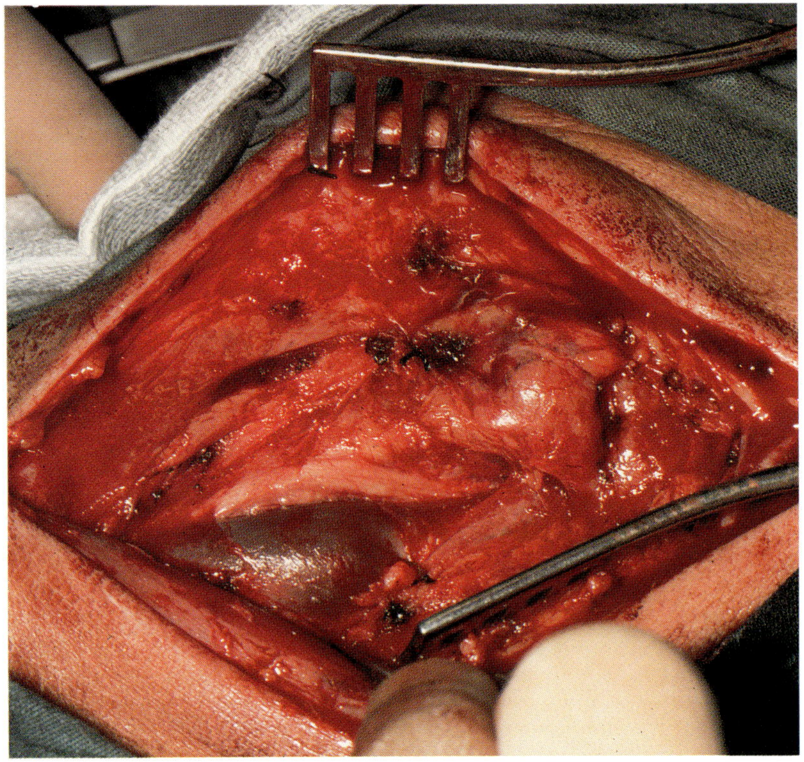

71

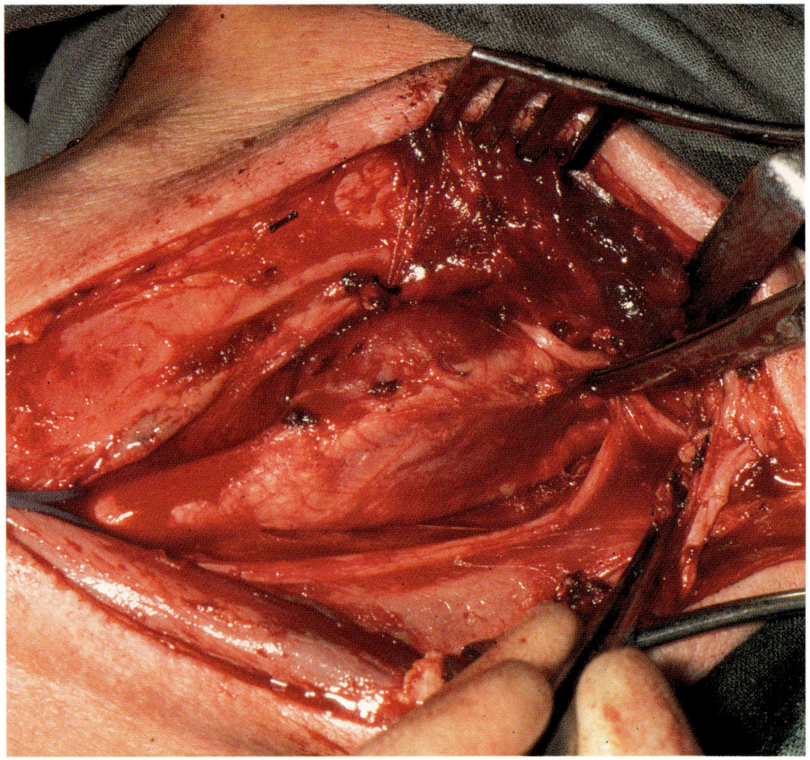

70 Further sharp dissection along the carotid sheath gives the first view of the common carotid, inferiorly. The upper carotid region is still covered by fibrofatty soft tissues containing small veins and lymph nodes, which are dissected free and sent for histological examination. Frozen section is not suitable for this material.

71 Having cleared these tissues from the upper carotid area the tumour and the external carotid artery are well exposed, with the hypoglossal nerve above and the vagus behind. The internal carotid can just be seen behind the tumour, in front of the vagus and internal jugular vein.

72

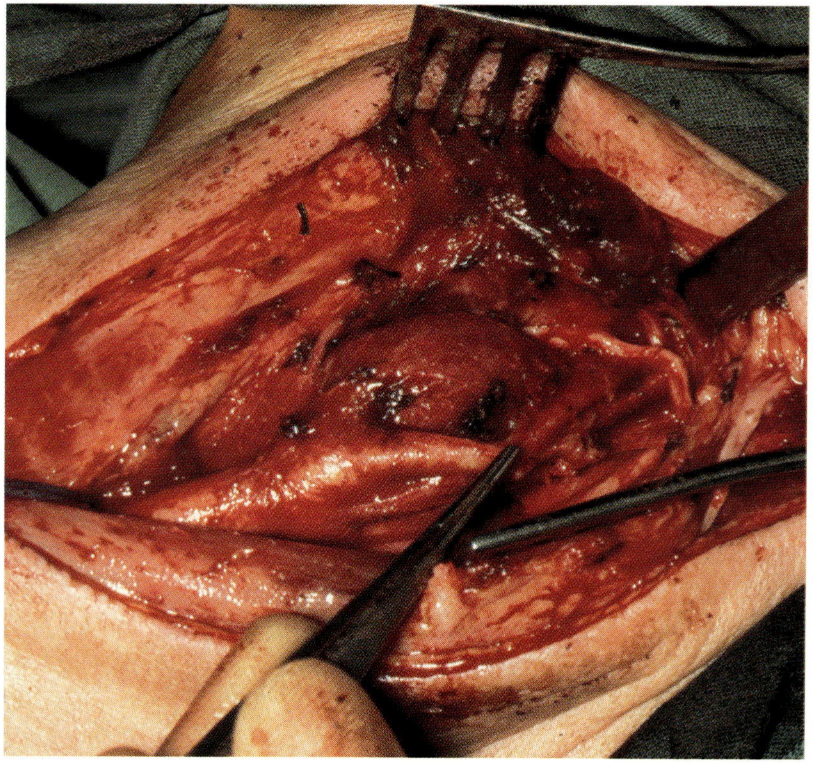

72 The plane of separation between the external carotid and the tumour is slowly and carefully developed and extended, using sharp dissection, just into the adventitia, with frequent pauses for the diathermy sealing of multiple fine bleeding points.

73

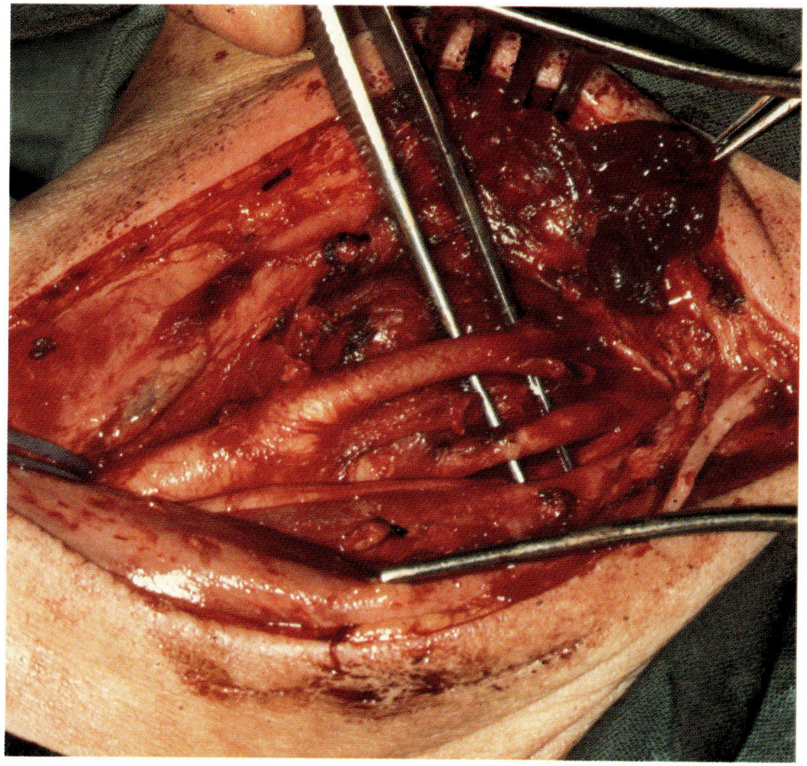

73 The internal carotid is now mobilised. There are many fewer vascular adhesions to the tumour, which can therefore be separated from the vessel much more easily. In this case it was possible to mobilise the tumour from above along both arteries.

74

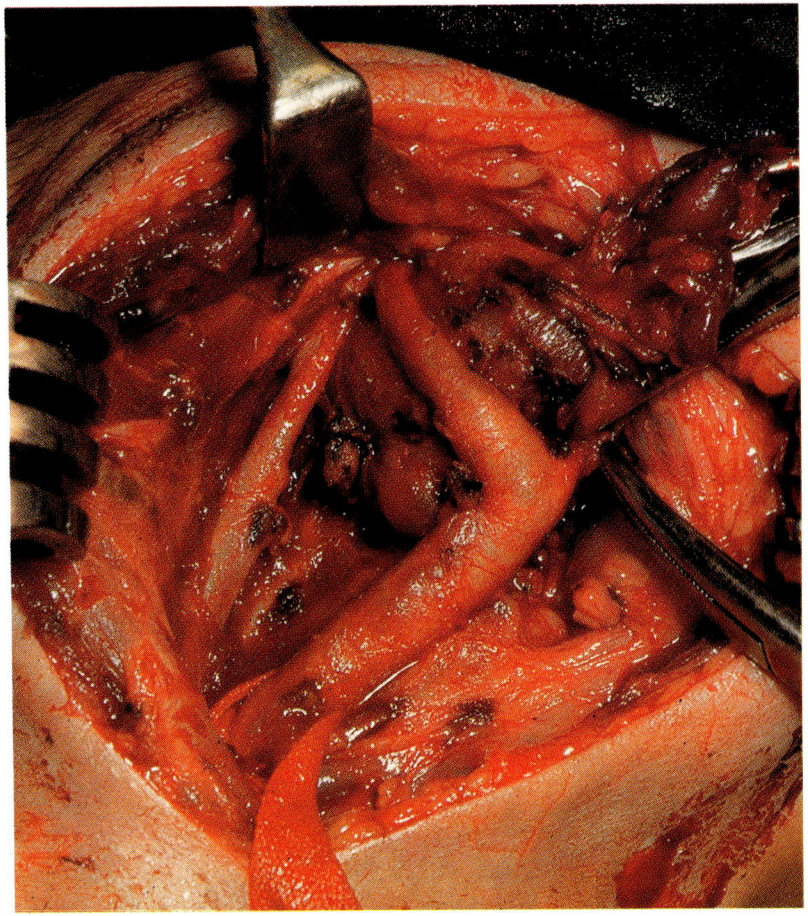

74 This is the tumour shown in Figure **60.** The external carotid may be difficult to free from the tumour in its proximal part, where most of the tumour supply arises. As the tumour lies deep to the artery, which may hold it down like a girdle, obscuring the internal carotid, the dissection at this stage can become hazardous. It is at this stage that the carotid may be entered (Figures **90** to **96** show such a case).

75

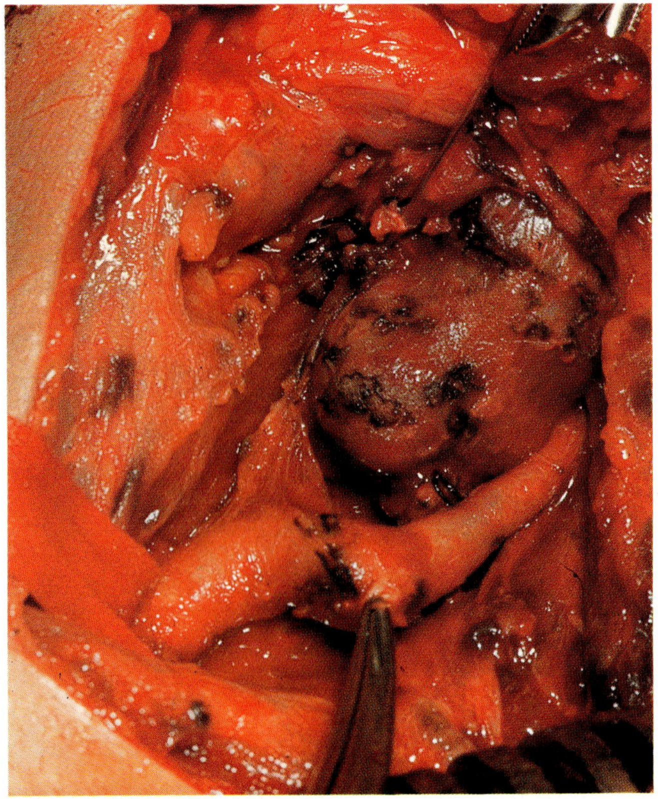

75 It is often helpful at this stage carefully to ligate the external carotid, not too close to its origin. This gives a safer exposure of the internal carotid and the whole lower part of the tumour, and of the most difficult phase of the proximal dissection. It is better to divide the external carotid than to enter the lumen at the bifurcation. The vessels behind the bifurcation having been secured the tumour can then be lifted up inferiorly and the easier phase of carotid separation upwards along the now freely visible internal carotid is completed. This muscular artery may be quite contracted at this stage (see also Figure **73**), which may account for the accident of its division during neck exploration for suspected malignant lymph nodes in cases explored without previous angiography.

The upper part of the tumour is gently freed from the hypoglossal nerve which may be displaced or even enveloped by the tumour. It may safely be dissected out of the now almost avascular tumour.

76

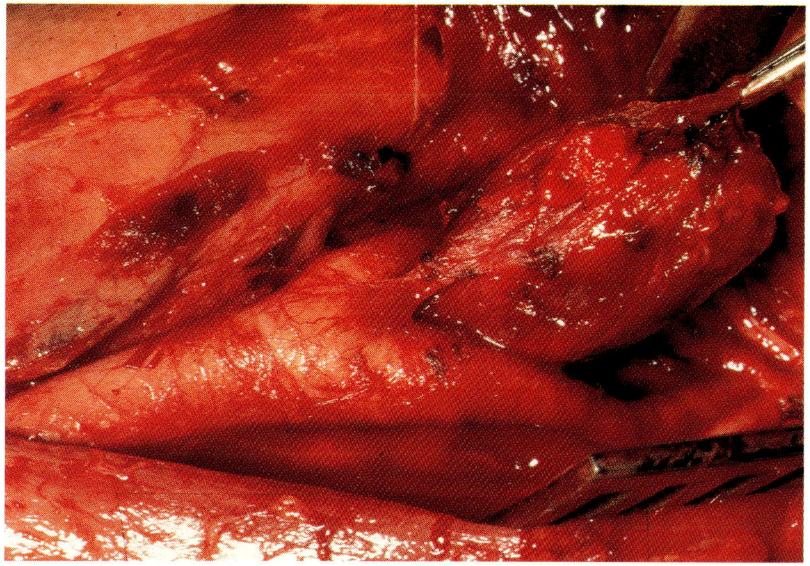

76 Returning to the first case, after the point reached in Figure **73**, the remaining lower portion of the internal carotid artery is freed from the tumour which may now be held up on its inter-carotid vascular pedicle, which is then secured by carefully placed ligatures. Fine vascular sutures may also be required for the shorter vessels.

78

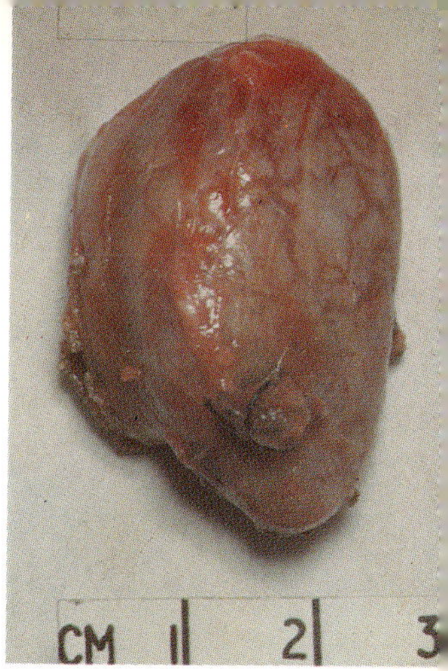

78 The excised tumour (case 2) retains a smooth contour and grooves from the carotids are seen over its lower portion.

77

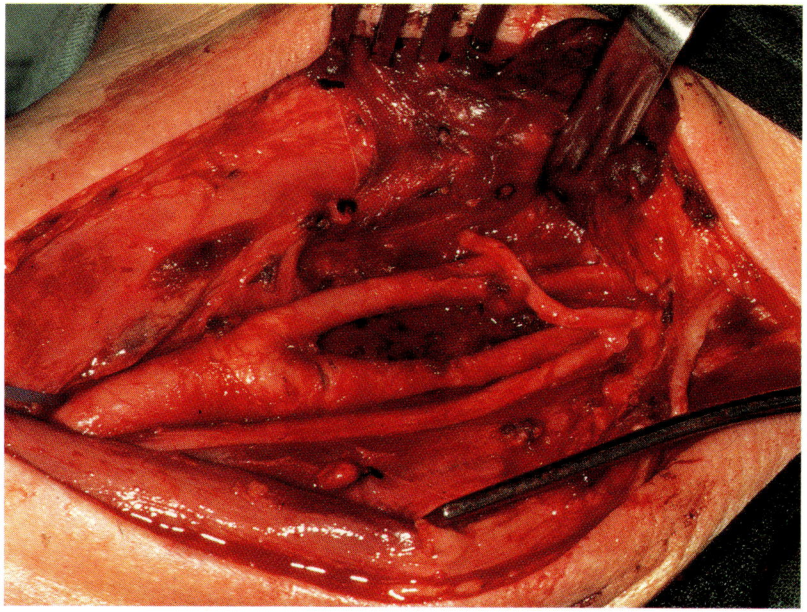

77 After removal of the tumour the carotids lie almost parallel. Wound closure is as for end-arterectomy (Figures **55** to **59**). There is no special after care for these patients, who are not at stroke risk if the carotids have not required clamping or repair.

Hazards and mishaps

If the carotid is entered, then vascular clamping with a light clamp such as Dardik's will be necessary. Fine vascular repair sutures will be required, and in exceptional circumstances a saphenous vein graft. In this event a carotid shunt should be inserted and the patient is heparinised. Division of the hypoglossal nerve or the vagus should be made good by accurate suture repair.

A case of false aneurysm of the carotid bifurcation following carotid body tumour excision is shown in Figures **90** to **96**.

Excision of internal carotid aneurysm

Like carotid body tumours, these are uncommon and chiefly affect women, though usually of an older age group. They are also silent clinically at first, but have a very real potential for causing embolic stroke, either spontaneously or during operative removal.

79

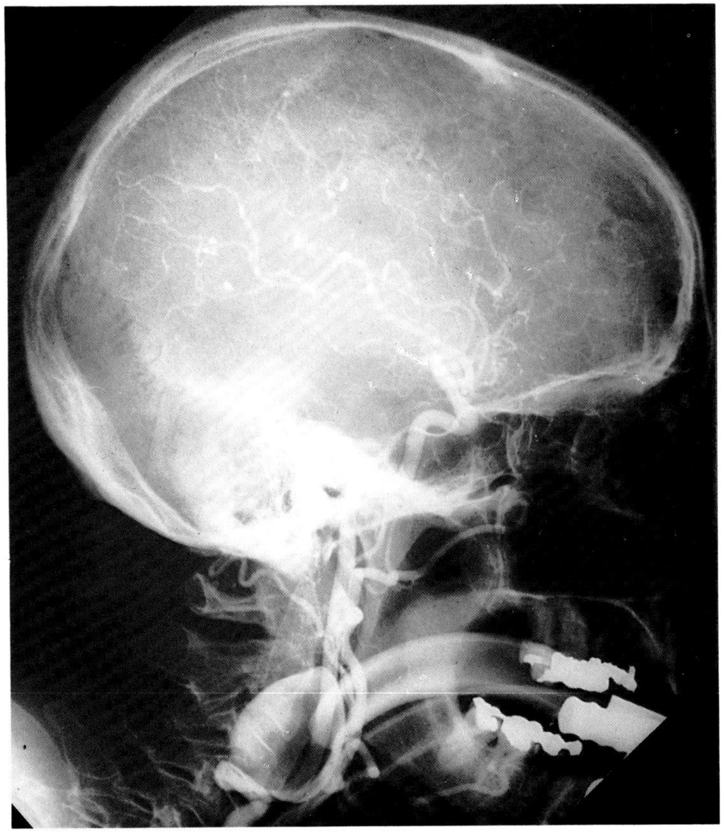

80

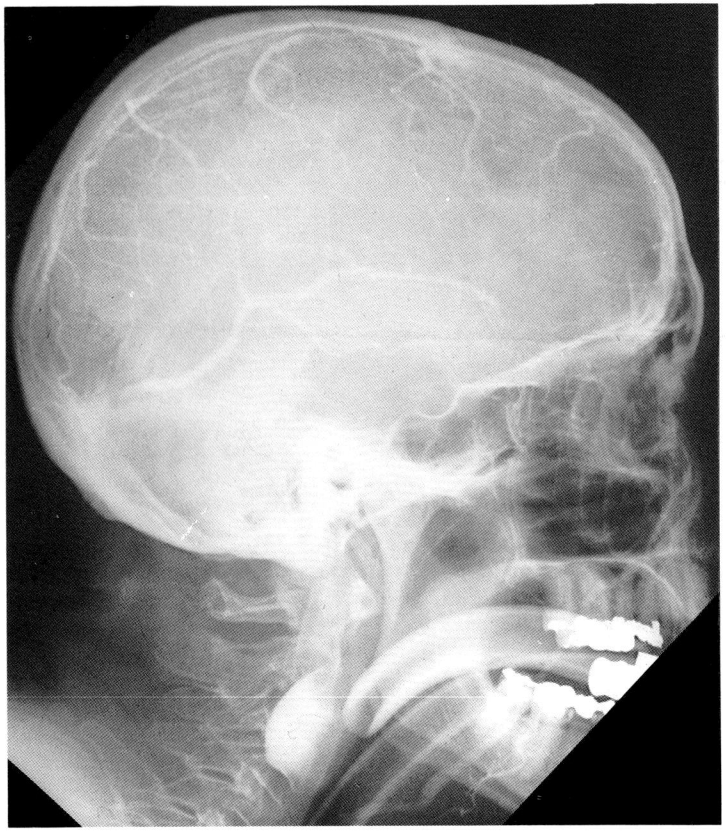

79 Selective right carotid arteriogram, showing a 3cm internal carotid aneurysm in a kinked and elongated artery. The patient was a woman aged 52 in good general health.

80 Delayed arteriogram film showing contrast medium lingering in the sac at a time when the main bolus has reached the cerebral veins.

81

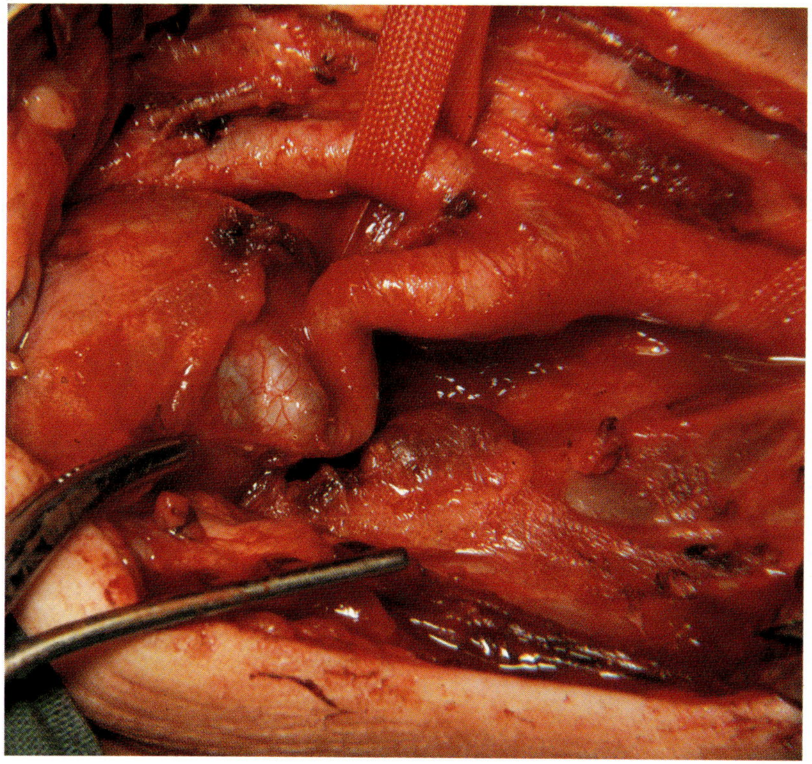

81 Exposure of the carotid bifurcation shows the kinked nature of the internal carotid leading to the lower part of the aneurysm, lying much higher in the neck than the arteriogram had suggested. The common and external carotids have been taped.

82

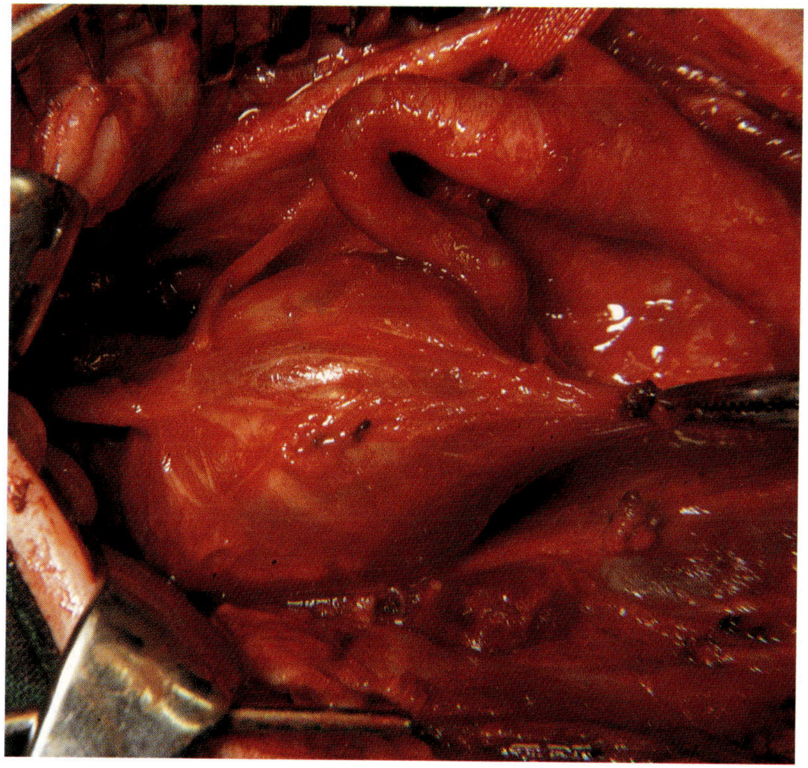

82 The sac is gently drawn down into the wound by its loose outer layers. It is *never* to be grasped or compressed at this stage. The distal internal carotid can now be seen, also the hypoglossal nerve.

83

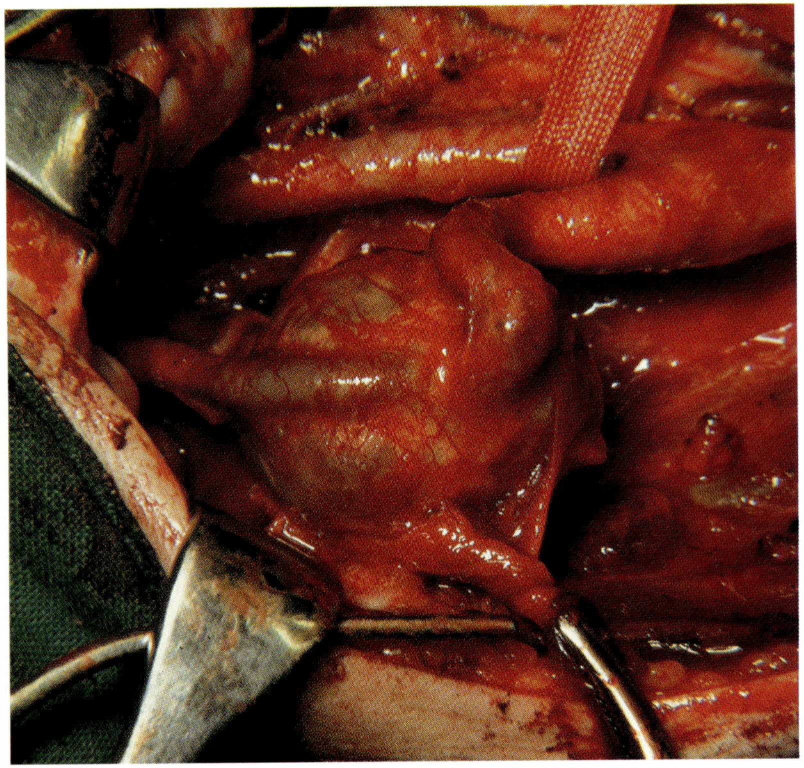

84

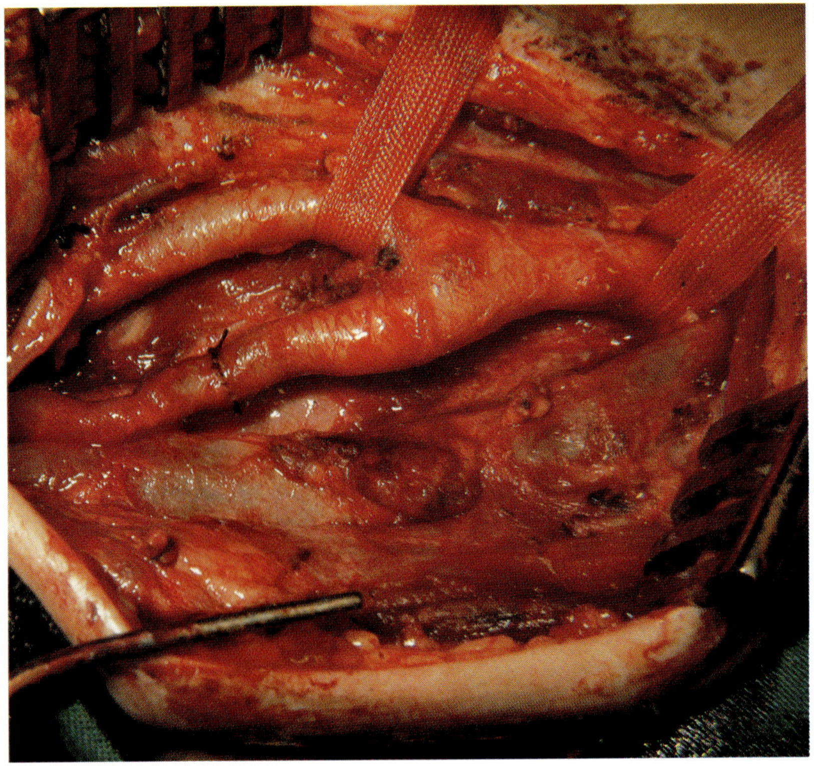

83 Careful further dissection of the distal internal carotid with the aneurysm still held down carefully. Distal control by means of a silastic loop or light arterial clamp will now allow a more normal manipulation of the sac and nearby vessels without risk of embolisation.

84 Resection with end to end anastomosis with 6/0 polypropylene completes the procedure. Drain and closure as in Figures **55** to **59.**

85

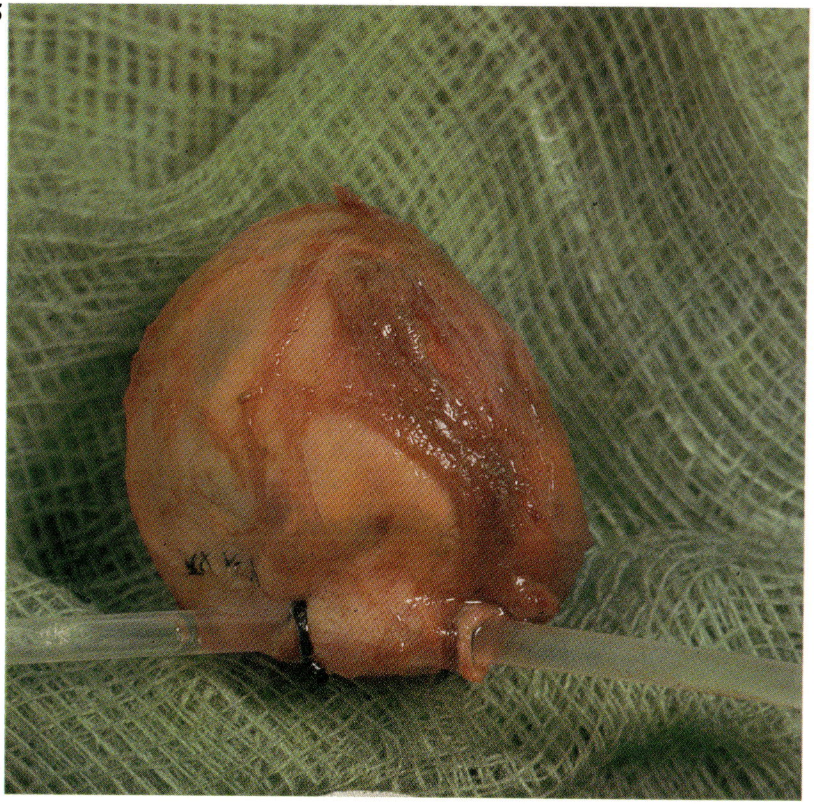

85 The excised sac with short segment of internal carotid. This condition may be a form of fibromuscular arterial dysplasia, and like it may be associated with intracranial aneurysms. The cerebral phase of carotid arteriography should always therefore be studied carefully in such cases.

Internal carotid ligation for cervical aneurysm

86

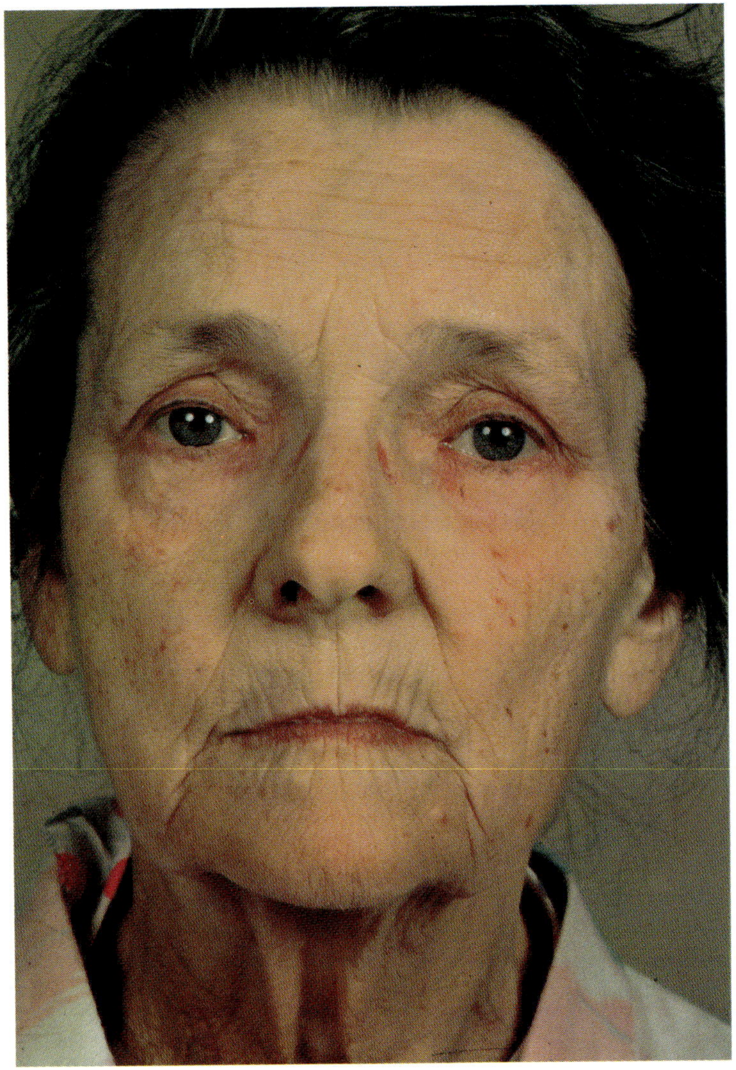

87

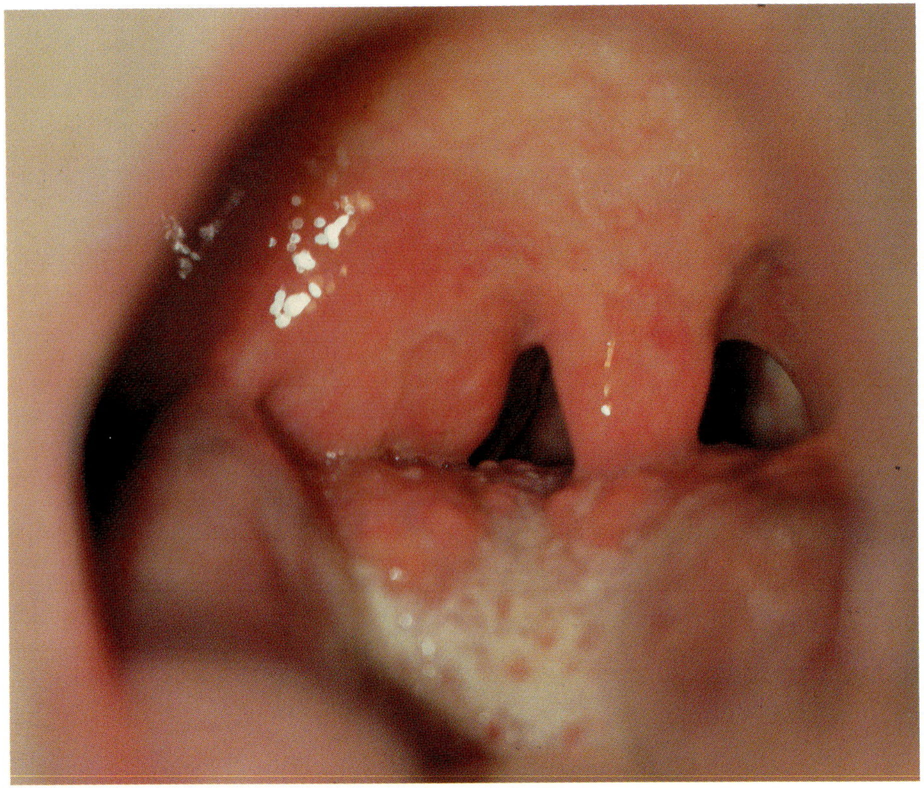

86 & 87 This elderly lady, whose facies suggests scleroderma, was found to have a pulsatile right retrotonsillar swelling that at first sight suggested a quinsy. Another of the author's patients, a child aged 2½ was referred with a pack in place to control the bleeding after an incision had been made with this diagnosis as its basis.

88

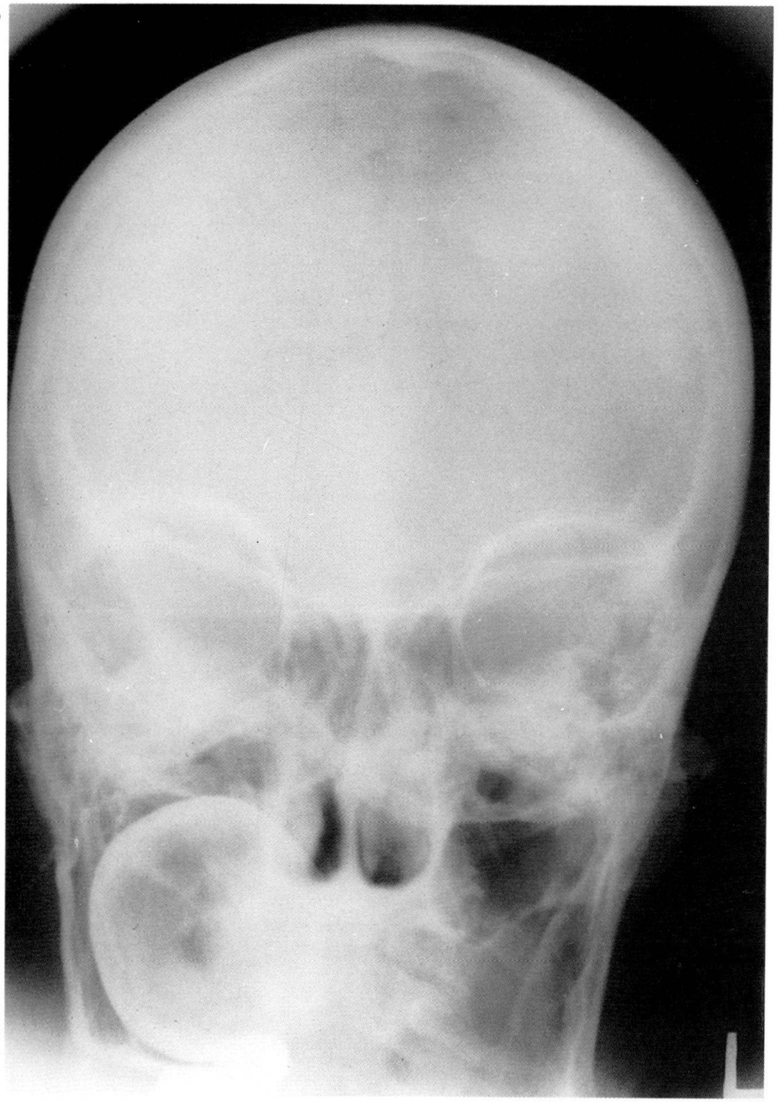

88 Anteroposterior carotid arteriography confirmed the extremely high position of this sac (compare Figures **79** and **80**).

89

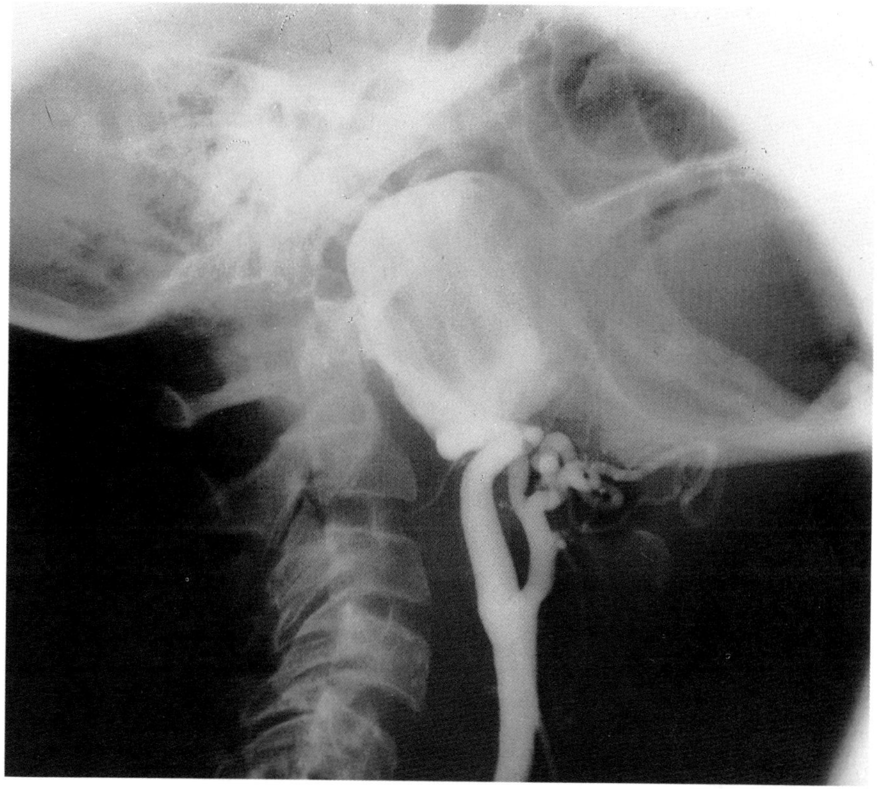

89 Lateral view of this arteriogram shows the same kinked appearance as in the younger woman in the earlier case.

At operation the normal bifurcation was exposed and the stump pressure of the internal carotid was over 80cm. Trial clamping produced no change in a cerebral activity monitor, so the internal carotid artery was ligated. The patient made a good recovery.

Repair of false aneurysm of carotid bifurcation

90

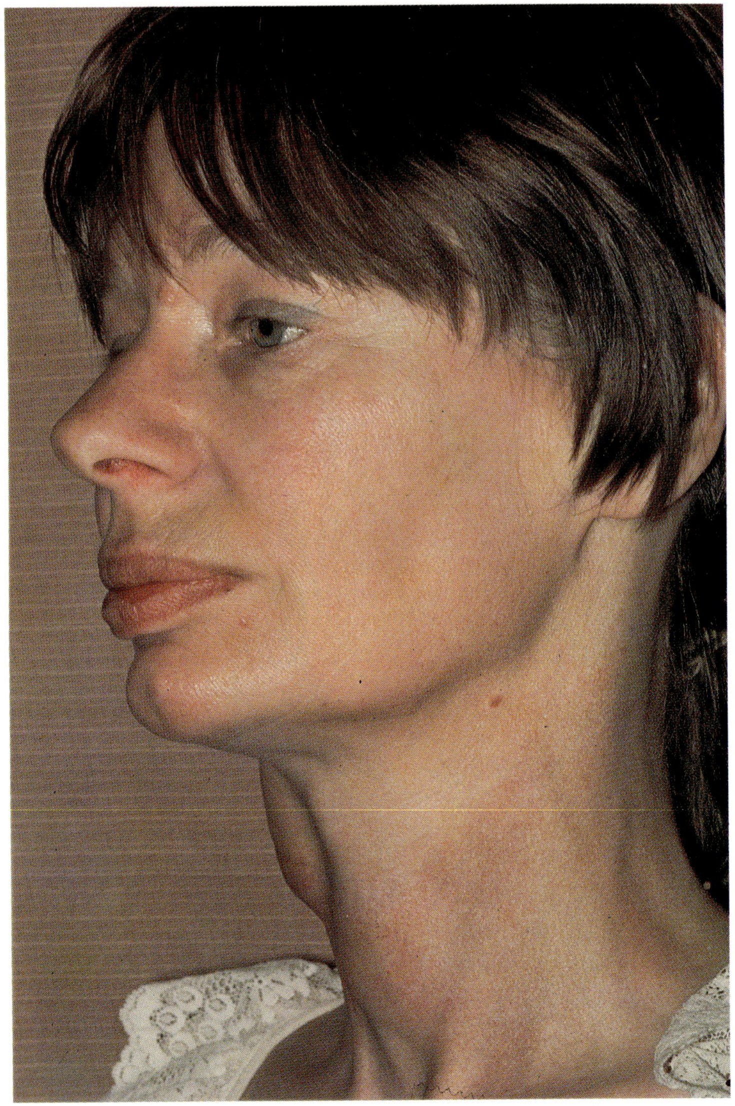

91

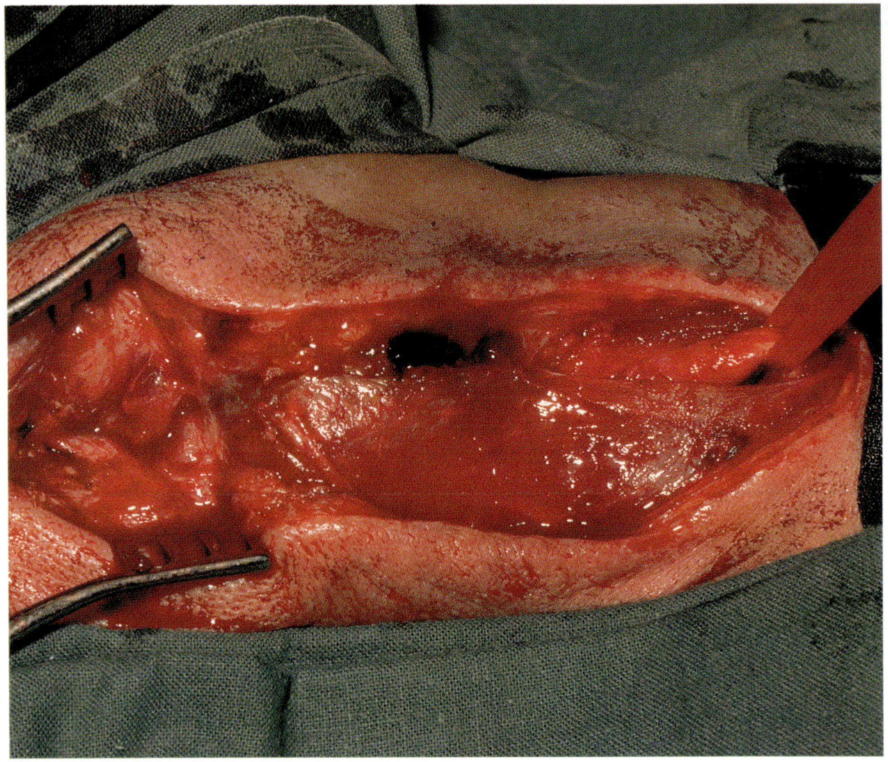

90 This lady aged 48 was referred with an expanding, pulsatile mass in the right carotid triangle, three weeks after a carotid body tumour had been excised. There had been bleeding problems at the first operation.

91 At operation the aneurysmal clot was found to have reached the subcutaneous layer of the neck. As with all false aneurysms, the first step was to secure the main arterial inflow, by taping the common carotid.

92

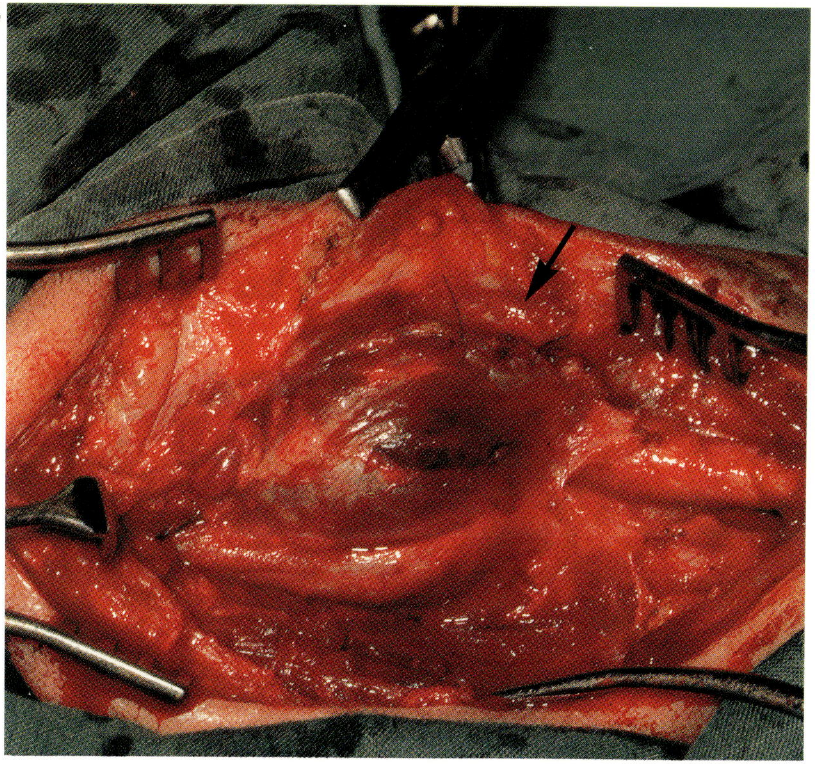

92 The internal carotid was then cautiously traced over the false sac up to a point at which it became free from it. Note sutures of previous operation (arrow).

93

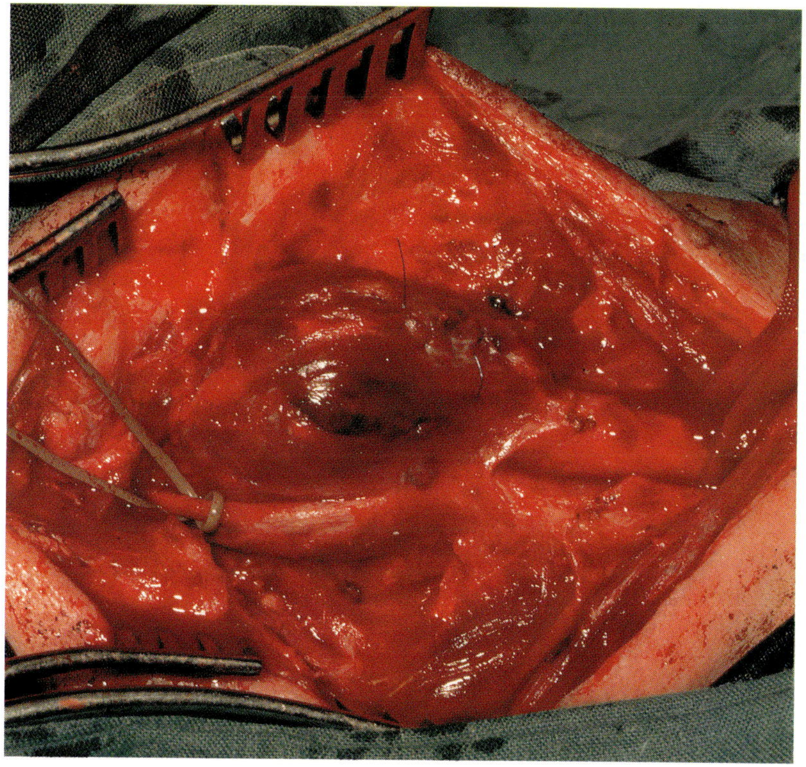

93 The distal internal carotid could then be secured with a silastic loop, to allow further mobilisation of the carotid bifurcation and its aneurysm, without risk of cerebral embolism.

94

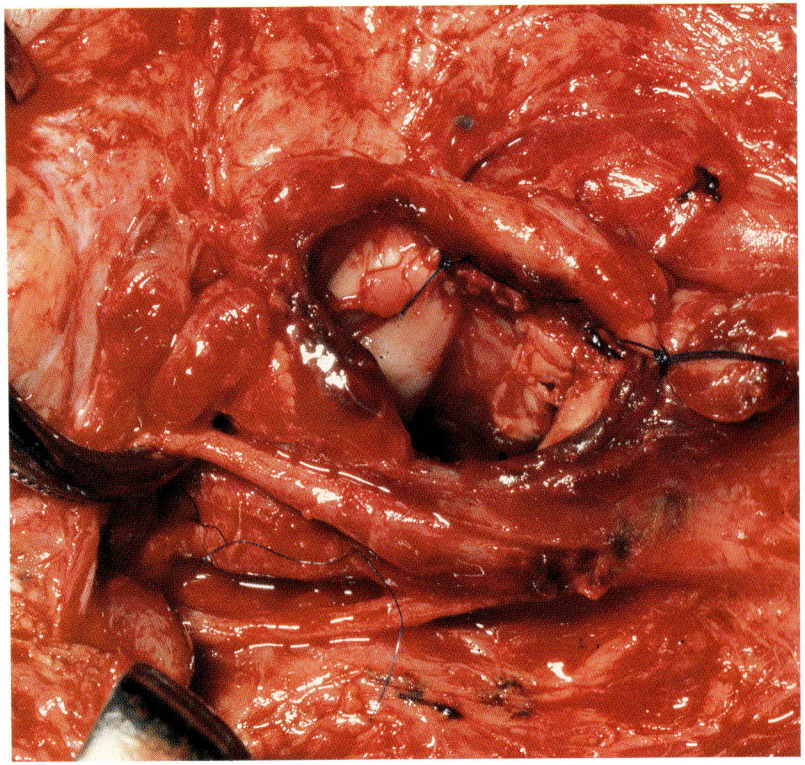

95

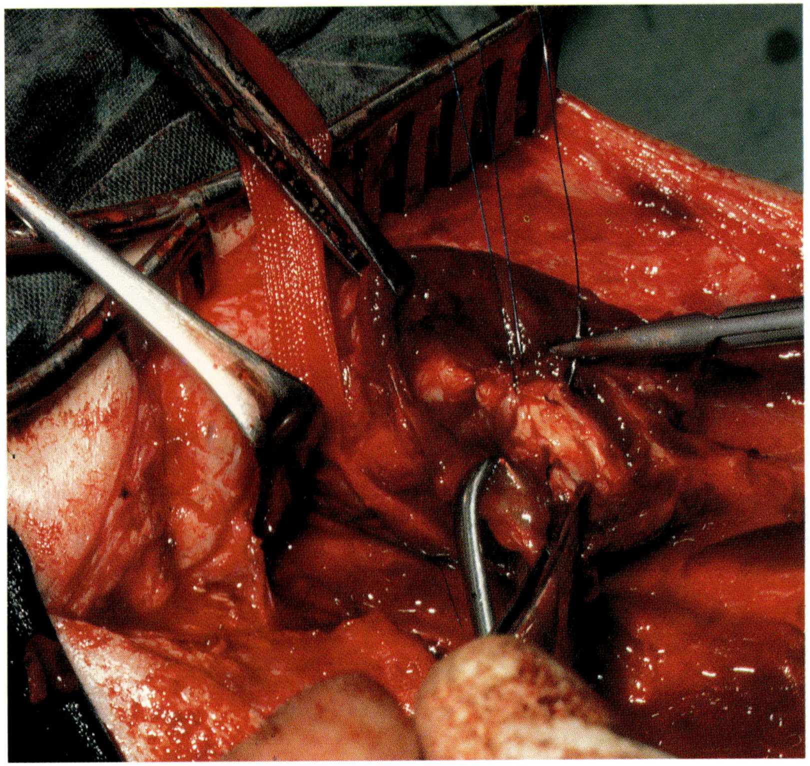

94 With all three carotids occluded the sac was opened. A previous suture line can be seen. Note the small size of the distal internal carotid, which is typical of this muscular artery during operative manipulation.

95 Simple suture of the long defect with 4/0 polypropylene was possible, as shown in the line drawing (Figure **96**). With the measured stump pressure at 120 cm no shunt was needed.

96

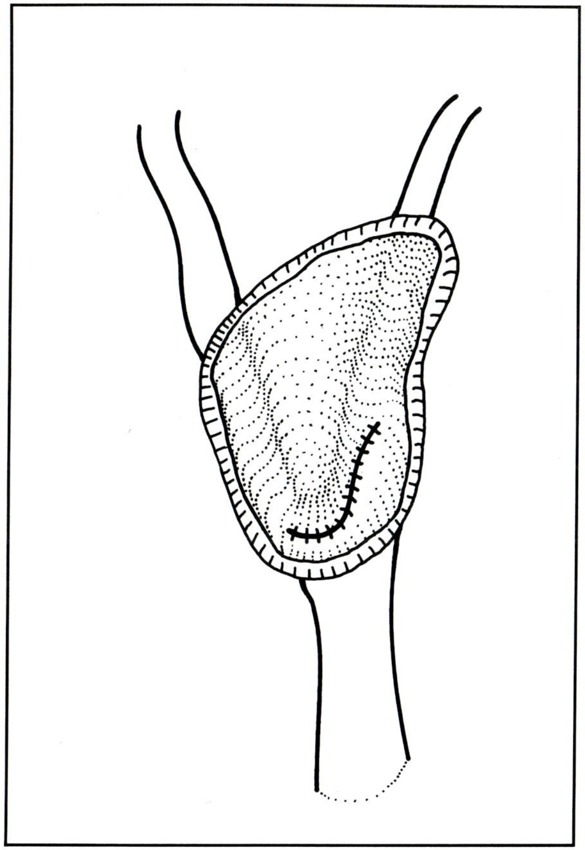

96 The defect in the carotid bifurcation occupied the site of major vascular adherence to the external carotid (see Figures **61** and **74** to **76**). Had the arterial tissues been unable to support the tension of simple suture, a venous patch graft from the ankle would have been used.

Other types of cervical carotid aneurysm

97

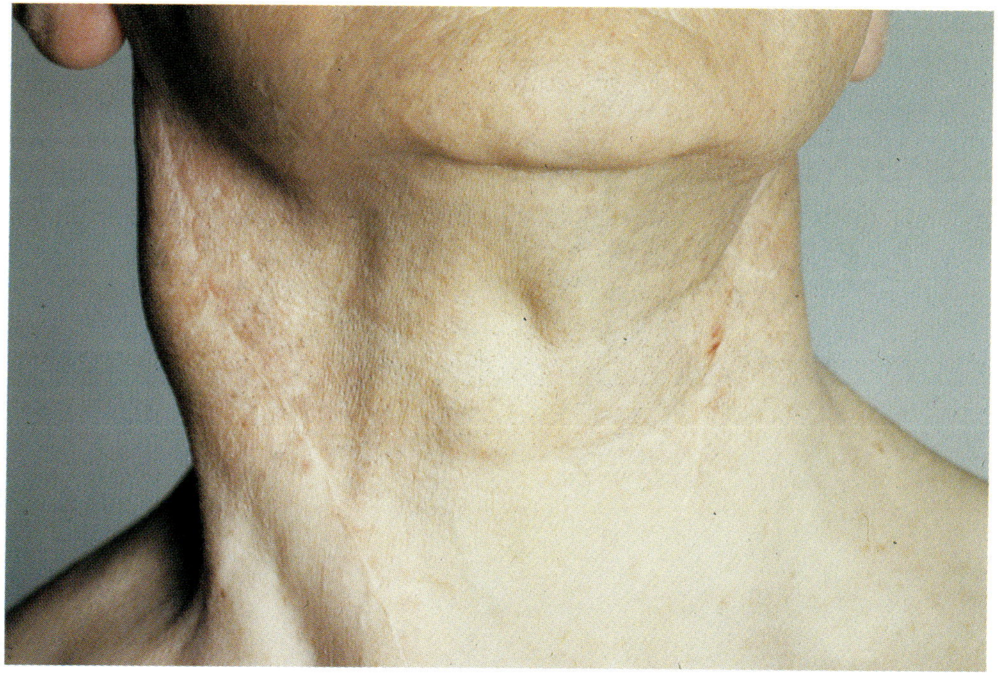

97 This patient had undergone carotid endarterectomy on both sides; on the left with simple suture, the normal practice with most vascular surgeons; though on the right it had been thought necessary to use a knitted dacron patch to avoid narrowing of the repair. Three years later he presented with a pulsatile swelling under the centre of the scar on this side, which at operation proved to be a fibrous false aneurysm with the patch forming a small part of its wall. Repair by venous patching was satisfactory.

98

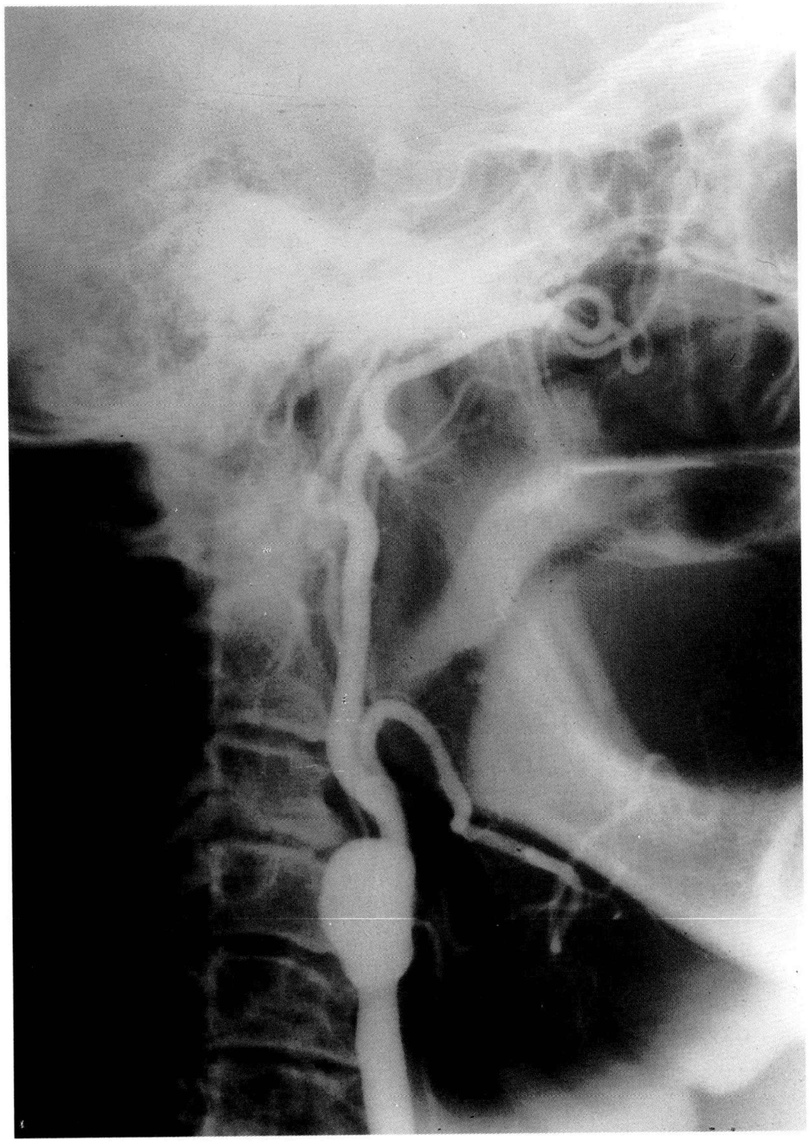

98 Another man whose right internal carotid had occluded without clinical effects at some time after his carotid endarterectomy developed this aneurysmal widening of the lower arteriotomy line which has not, however, progressed. It may represent the fusiform dilatation often seen in an endarterectomised segment with prolonged late patency. Subsequent major neck surgery for pharyngeal carcinoma was completed without vascular problems.

99

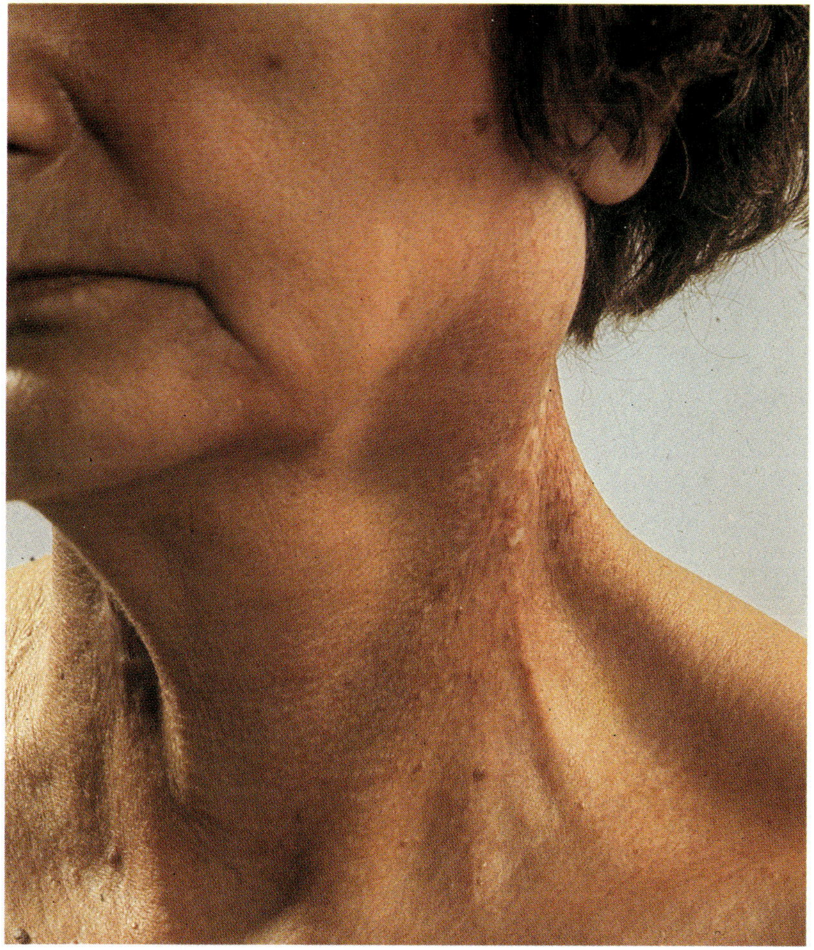

99 A lady of 70 presented with a large pulsatile left carotid swelling at the site of X-irradiation of tuberculous lymph nodes in her childhood.

100

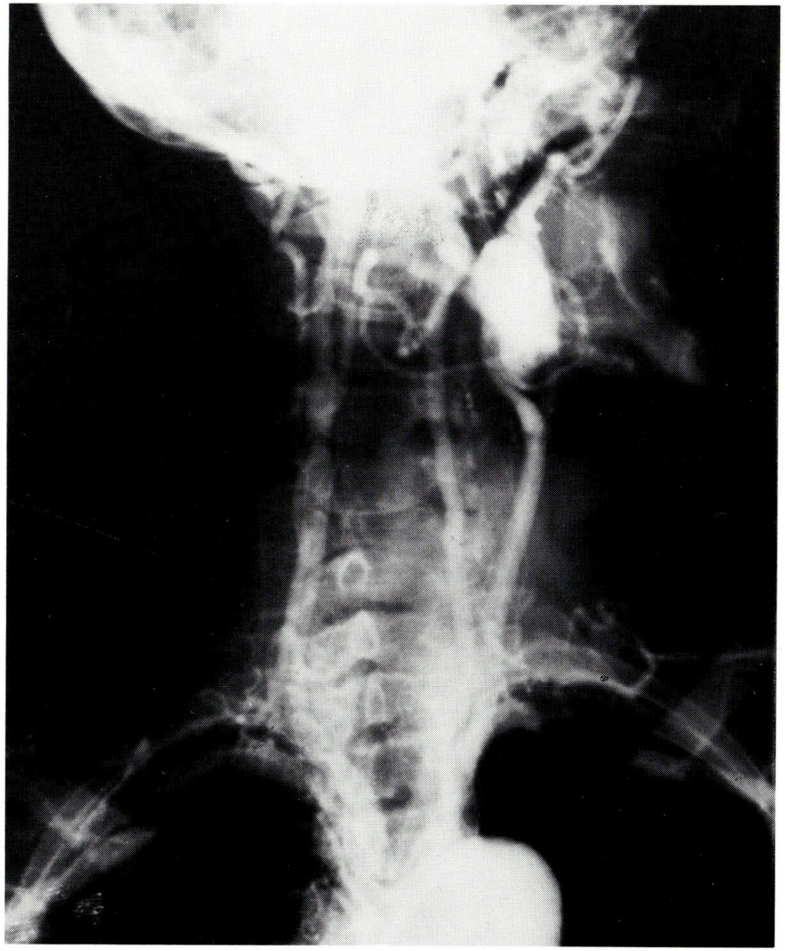

100 Arch aortography showed a large saccular aneurysm of the internal carotid, which was subsequently excised and replaced with a saphenous vein graft.

Conclusion

The surgery of the internal carotid is almost always attended by concern over the sufficiency of the cerebral blood supply. Careful handling of the artery at operation, and the knowledge that stump pressure is sufficient should avoid the occurrence of operative stroke. Good care during recovery ensures uneventful recovery in those who reach this stage neurologically intact.

Further reading

Angell-James, J.E. and Lumley, J.S.P. (1974) The effects of carotid endarterectomy on the mechanical properties of the carotid sinus and carotid sinus nerve activity in atherosclerotic patients. *British Journal of Surgery,* **61,** 805–810.

Bernstein, E.F., Humber, P.B., Collins, G.M., Dilley, R.B., Devin, J.B. and Hart, S.H. (1983) Life expectancy and late stroke following carotid endarterectomy. *Annals of Surgery,* **198,** 80–86.

Dehn, T.C.B., and Taylor, G.W. (1983) Cranial and cervical nerve damage associated with carotid endarterectomy. *British Journal of Surgery,* **70,** 365–368.

Eastcott, H.H.G. (1976) Surgical management of carotid and vertebral occlusive disease. In: *Stroke. Proceedings of the Ninth Pfizer International Symposium.* (pp 458–468.) Churchill Livingstone, Edinburgh.

Lees, C.D., Levine, H.L., Beven, E.G. and Tucker, H.M. (1981) Tumours of the carotid body. Experience with 41 cases. *American Journal of Surgery,* **142,** 362–365.

McCollum, C.H., Wheeler, W.G., Noon, G.P. and DeBakey, M.E. (1979) Aneurysms of the extracranial carotid artery. *American Journal of Surgery,* **137,** 196–200.

Sundt, T.M., Sandok, B.A. and Whisnant, J.P. (1975) Carotid endarterectomy. Complications and preoperative assessment of risk. *Mayo Clinic Proceedings,* **50,** 301–306.

Thompson, J.E. (1976) Carotid surgery for cerebrovascular insufficiency. *Current Problems in Surgery,* **15,** 5–68.

Index

All numbers refer to pages